# MAD COWS
## and
# MILK GATE

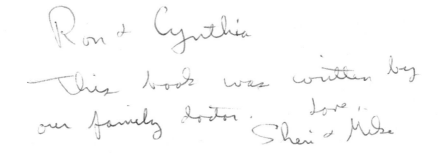

*Ron & Cynthia*
*This book was written by*
*our family doctor.*
*Love,*
*Sheri & Mike*

# VIRGIL HULSE M.D., MPH, FACPM

Marble Mountain Publishing

# Virgil Hulse, M.D., MPH, FACPM

Additional copies are available. For your convenience, an order form can be found at the back of this book.

PRINTED IN THE UNITED STATES OF AMERICA
by
MARBLE MOUNTAIN PUBLISHING
P.O. Box 668
Phoenix, Oregon 97535


Library of Congress Catalog Card Number: 96-78006
ISBN 0-9654377-0-1

## COMMENTS

"Thoroughly documented and equally "disturbing this powerful book takes you back to the enormous health advantages of a more plantfood centered diet." "Reading this book is a matter of Life and death." "A powerful eye opener." "Just as Watergate changed the course of history, so Milkgate is destined to change the course of our diet. If we don't, God help us!" Dr. Hans Diehl, Lifestyle medicine Institute, Loma Linda, Ca. Author, Epidemiologist, Nutritionist.

I have followed the career of the author of this book since 1948. We agree on fundamental concerns, the welfare of our patients and those who seek our advice deserve the very best that we can give for their health and happiness. Great changes have taken place in the dairy industry in the past half century. The cows have gone from a total vegetarian cow to a flesh-eating animal.

Dr. Virgil Hulse has lived during the time of these major changes. First hand, starting as a dairy worker, then to inspector, and then as a physician, he has closely followed this transition. His background and training allows him to piece together the cause and effect of these changes in the marked increase in diseases of the cow. His honesty and concerns compels him to speak out clearly. Why? The next problem we face, physicians and others, will be a major increase in the diseases of the human, unless we make appropriate changes brought out in this book. Cow's milk is known to be a major component in the cause of certain degenerative diseases such as allergies, atherosclerosis, arthritis, and type-1 diabetes. We had reason enough to give up animal milks for food before the problems of infectious agents. Perhaps now the public will change and be relieved of many of these other ailments as they give up milk products. Milton Crane, M.D. Newstart Medical Clinic, Weimar Institute, Weimar, Ca.

"Mad Cows and Milk Gate" serves as a reminder that we must be alert to the fact that our food supply has the potential to be a serious problem for our general health. Reading the book will not only heighten ones awareness of the problem but also allow one to make personal choices to their own food consumption. Gerald B. Ahmann, MD, Ph.D., Hemotologist-Oncologist

"For decades Dr. Hulse has taken a courageous and firm position regarding the significant health hazards of dairy products. This book not only provides a synopsis of his valuable work but also a driving incentive for the reader to make personal health behavioral changes and pass the work on to the unsuspecting!" Don Hoffman, Dr PH, Certified Health Education Specialist, San Bernardino, Calif.

I turned off the Olympics, sequestered myself in my room, and read Mad Cows and Milk Gate cover to cover, virtually without putting it down. At first I was skeptical of these topics and obviously we need a lot more research and answers, but I was thoroughly impressed with your dedication to these topics and your unique vantage point, given your background, If only 1% of what you fear is true, world society is in a much bigger fix than simply what we know already about this Pandora's box. Since reading your book, I have personally decided to stay away from dairy products until I have more time to think about the risk/benefit ratio of using dairy products. I have a great fear of mutant prions invading this country given our insane practices of bovine cannibalism.

Your contribution to society in terms of your book is impressive. You've done a lot of work, over a long time, and, from your background, can provide unique insight into these issues. Congratulations, I'm sure that society will benefit greatly from all your hard work and perspicacity. John A. Walker M.D. Gastroenterologist Medford, Oregon 97504

Dr. Hulse has provided us with an authoritative account of the current public health dangers in the dairy and beef industries. I commend him for his courage and expertise. I hope that the developers of public policy will show similar courage in placing the health of the American people above the economics of big industry. Ronald L. Peters, MD, MPH

## ACKNOWLEDGMENT

My deep appreciation and gratitude go to Betty, Angela, Elisabeth, Dana, Dean and Ethel. Who unfailingly and with a wonderful sense of humor listened, typed, proofed, encouraged and corrected. Thank you!
I also wish to acknowledge the interest and encouragement given to me by Marjorie Baldwin M.D., John McDougal M. D., Internist, author and T.V. personality, Milton Crane M.D. of the Wiemar Institute, California, and Yanto Lunardi-Iskandar M.D. of the National Institutes of Health.

## DEDICATION

I wish to dedicate this book to the many honest and ethical, research scientists around the world, who are working diligently to unlock the information about retroviruses.

# TABLE OF CONTENTS

# INTRODUCTION

It will all blow over. So our milk is dangerous--what's next? Should we stay home to avoid walking under a falling piano? Mad cow disease has been folded, stacked, slipped into news delivery bags, and hurled at the doors of suburban America. It's easy to view this breakthrough of information as a media gimmick that will die down. However, I can witness to the fact that this is not a gimmick, and the danger, if not the hype, will not blow over.

When the mad cow came out in the news the one word in my head was "Finally." I have been researching this problem now for 20 years. The rooms of my home and medical office are filled with papers, magazines, correspondences, and bills that have detailed the struggle since the late 70's. The case of the mad cow has not been exaggerated in the press, in fact, in many cases, the situation is much worse than has been told. Cows are being fed diseased sheep, chickens, and other cows. These cows are then slaughtered, wrapped in plastic, priced and put out in your local grocery store as harmless for human consumption. Of these cows, 80% have the bovine leukemia virus and 50% have the bovine immunodeficiency virus -- the animal equivalent of AIDS. We are drinking milk and eating cheese with lymphocytes that are loaded with the proviral DNA of these viruses. It is only common sense that when consuming a fluid that has been emitted from an animal, or the actual flesh itself, we the consumers, are at risk for whatever ailed the animal. The implications of this suggestion are so enormous that the dairy and meat industries have clung to the idea that it has not been proven that the species barrier could be crossed. As a doctor who has practiced for 30 years, this front impresses me about as much as a plastic dam sent to hold back all the fury of the ocean.

Many studies have been conducted which more than suggest that these diseases can infect humans as a result of eating milk or meat from diseased animals. In order for epidemiology studies to be fully credible a control group is needed. This is impossible with BLV and BIV because nearly everyone has consumed dairy products. However, recent mapping of the human genome has enabled us to see that ten percent of the genome has been invaded with retroviruses; viruses which come from animals.

Many have underestimated the danger of these retroviruses, trusting pasteurization, limited exposure, and a generally healthy diet to foolproof them from the disease in the food industries. In reality, it only takes one retrovirus to invade a body. My son was a victim of Hodgkin's disease. I am a victim of multiple myeloma. Our diets were saturated with milk products. I believe that retroviruses played a part in our pain and struggle. Retroviruses can be hosted inactively in our body for years. When our immune system is attacked by other viruses, toxic substances, or radiation, the cell that the virus is in may start replicating uncontrollably: overtaking an organ or an entire body with cancer cells.

I want to know why our government passed the Delaney Act and then does little to nothing about the scandals in the dairy industry. I want to know why our government passed this act that says products proven to cause cancer in testing animals can not be sold to the public and then ignores the tests that have been done. I want to know why our government as a ' world leader' has lagged shamefully behind many European countries when they refused to sell beef or milk from diseased cows and set up programs to end the problem.

No, the mad cow is not a sensational journalism gimmick. When cows in Great Britain are slaughtered in huge numbers because they are diseased something is seriously wrong. When cows which can no longer be sold or milked as in Britain become makeshift billboards for Ben and Jerry's ice cream- we should take notice.

But how? We have to go to work, rush home through traffic, make the kids dinner and drop exhausted in our beds. Relaxed days at the beach have gifted our skin with irreversible skin damage, our nuclear power plants could fail at any moment, our walls are made of asbestos and if that doesn't get us first we're receiving harmful radiation from our microwaves and computer screens daily. We may get cancer from our beef and milk? The weary consumer drones "Add it to the list."

The passive attitude of the American public seems to be what the dairy and meat industries have counted on. It's easy to feel that we can't do or change anything. But we are the people-- we are the government-- and we are the victims of unsafe standards. It is not outlandish to believe that our dairy and meat industries can be cleaned up, it has been done in many other countries. This is a step which has already been tested and laid out for America-- all we must do is take it.

My interest in the dairy industry first began in 1952 when I was a milk inspector. Since then I went to medical school, had five kids, and practiced medicine for 30 years. I have experience as a pasteurizer, milk and cream tester, buttermaker, ice cream maker, milk plant supervisor, and Dairy Herd Improvement Association Cow Tester. I received a Bob Hope California Dairy Industry Advisory Board Scholarship to attend Polytechnic College at San Luis Obispo where I received a Bachelor of Science degree in Agriculture in Dairy Manufacturing. I was a milk inspector for the State of Californian, counties of Fresno, San Francisco, Marin, Sonoma, Mendocino, Orange, and San Bernardino. I received a Master in Public Health degree in Environmental Health in Milk and Food Technology at the University of Michigan that was funded by a United States Public Health Traineeship. I received a M.D. degree from Loma Linda University. I then did post doctoral studies at the School of Public Health at Loma Linda University, and obtained a Master of Public Health degree in Cancer Epidemiology that was funded by a United States Public Health Traineeship. I was an Associate Professor of Family Practice at the School of Medicine at Loma Linda University. At present I am a member of the Retrovirus Committee of the United State Animal Health Association. I am board certified in Family Practice and also board certified in Preventive Medicine and Public Health. I am a Fellow of the American College of Preventive Medicine. I have practiced Family Medicine for thirty years and have an active licenses to practice medicine in the states of Oregon and California.

Currently I have taken a sabbatical from my practice to get this news to the public. I have watched with horror as my patients have died prematurely from cancer. One out of two men, and one out or three women will get an invasive cancer in their lifetime. What happened to the other people who did not get cancer? They died of other diseases which ended in heart attacks, strokes or infection. There are many diseases and evils in life that we can't do anything about. Thankfully this is not one of them. The National Cancer Institute has stated that cancer is probably related to our diet and environmental toxic substances. I have served my patients and my family and believe that the problems in the inspection standards have been major factors in their health and the health of all Americans.

Strangely, we have not given these problems the consideration or worry with which we treat such issues as the use of pesticides. Tragically, this problem is much worse because its path is unknown. Prions, which cause mad cow disease, are a totally new infectious agent. Prions cannot be killed at even 360 degrees C, and pasteurization levels are more in the neighborhood of 161 degrees F. It is not a bacteria, it is not a virus, and we are at risk because of its effects.

We don't have time for E. coli. We don't have time for salmonella. We don't have time to wonder if we're getting cancer or AIDS from our meat or our milk products. Certainly, all milk served to our children and adults should be free of the leukemia virus and produced from leukemia-free cows. Many European countries have taken decisive measures while we have sat idly by. What is our excuse? An eradication program such as the one employed in Europe would save millions in health costs. It appears that there is a conflict of interest that occurs in those agencies in our federal government that are responsible for food production and promotion and also public health and food inspection.

It is my purpose in writing this book that we will no longer be able to claim ignorance. I have faith that the American public will place more value on their health than the traditional regressive standards of the dairy and meat industries. I have faith that the American public will recognize the danger and pass the necessary laws for our basic survival.

The social-contract theory of our government, by which we pay taxes to earn protection must be upheld. We have not been attacked by a visibly aggressive enemy. We suffer from the risks of disease by an enemy that is part of nearly every household and every diet. As members of a free society we are not impotent. We the people, we the government, must claim our right to protection.

The decision to write this book was a difficult one made over a long period of time. I have great respect for many in the dairy industry, and I believe they have high ethical and sanitary standards. I believe our government agencies try hard to fulfill their dual roles of supporting the agricultural industry and protecting the health of the consumers. However, I do not believe they have seen the large overall picture; and the importance in this scenario of the newly developing infectious agents, viruses, mutants of viruses, and prions.

I have 30 years of practicing medicine and 44 years worth of involvement with the dairy industry in my wake. I want to share with you what I have seen. I want to give you an honest look at problems the average person doesn't know about but is affected by nonetheless. I have seen the issue from both sides and concluded that the health of the American public is in jeopardy.

# CHAPTER ONE

# MAD COWS

## GUESS WHAT'S COMING WITH DINNER

You sit down to your favorite dinner. Everything looks perfect. The trimmings are there. The beef is cooked just the way you like it. As the aroma drifts through your house, delighting your senses, it seems as though nothing could be amiss. But could you be getting more with this meal than you planned? After spending fifteen years as a milk inspector in the state of California, my interest is naturally aroused whenever I see or hear news reports about farm animals, particularly cattle. Of course, it would be impossible to mention everything that's been said about animal diseases. In this chapter I've included an overview of some of the most current studies. Appalling as this information may be, Americans need this awareness when choosing their nutritional intake.

## ANIMAL DISEASES ARE A MAJOR PROBLEM

Prior to 1980, prior to the AIDS 'epidemic' in man and the Mad Cow disease 'epidemic,' it was widely believed that infectious diseases were no longer much of a threat in the developed world. The remaining challenges to public and animal health, it was thought, stemmed from noninfectious diseases such as cancer, heart disease and degenerative diseases. That confidence was shattered by the AIDS epidemic and the Mad Cow disease in cattle.

Mad Cow disease is probably a new term to you, but in Great Britain it has made headlines and now all over the world. The fear that eating contaminated beef can lead to dementia and death has greatly decreased consumption of beef products. Mad Cow disease, technically known as bovine spongiform encephalopathy, or BSE, is a fatal degenerative disease affecting the central nervous system of cattle. It is similar to certain neurological diseases affecting humans.[1]

## MAD SHEEP DISEASE JUMPS TO CATTLE

The general assumption, accepted by the British Veterinary Association, is that cattle died of Mad Cow disease by eating meat and bone meal of sheep infected with a scrapie-like agent (scrapie is a neurological disease that affects sheep). The agent was not inactivated in the process of rendering and was incorporated into cattle feed in the form of meat and bone meal. Then the disease was further spread to cattle probably in the later stages by recycling of infected material from cattle.[2] As meal containing bits of infectious sheep was fed to cows, they may have developed BSE. As bits of these cows were then converted into meal and fed back to other cows, the disease spread. The chain of transmission continued as infected cattle were used as feed for other cows and animals.

Great Britain, with over 160,000 cases may be the worst but is certainly not the only country affected by BSE. The other countries and total reported cases are Guernsey, 524; Northern Ireland, 1,642; Jersey, 109; Isle of Man 375; Republic of Ireland, 102; Switzerland, 180; Portugal, 31; and France, 12. Countries which have had imported BSE cases only include Germany (4 cases), Canada (1), Denmark (1), Falkland Islands (1), Italy (2), and Oman (2).

As a result of the Mad Cow disease, Britain has taken a number of actions, including (1) prohibiting the inclusion of feeding cows ruminant-derive meat in all ruminant rations, (2) prohibiting the consumption of milk from suspect animals by either animals or humans, (3) stopping the use of certain bovine organs, such as brain, for human consumption, and (4) destroying all animals showing signs of BSE and indemnifying the owners.[3]

Also, since the transmission of the Mad Cow disease to humans is a subject of major concern throughout the United

Kingdom and Europe, a study has been initiated to monitor the incidence of human brain disorders over the coming years. Mad Cow disease has never been diagnosed in the U.S. but spongiform encephalopathy or Scrapie (Mad Sheep) in sheep is widespread in the U.S. and is increasing rapidly. Meat and bone meal from ruminates is used extensively in cattle rations throughout the U.S. over the last five years, it has become common in milking herd rations.[4]

## POTENTIAL FOR TRANSMISSION TO HUMANS

I believe there is a high, unexplored potential for transmission of Mad Cow disease to humans. The basic rationale in support of this position assumes that some change or mutation in the scrapie agent permitted it to infect cattle and the modified agent has greater potential to cross other species barriers. Cattle, mice, sheep, goats and pigs have died as a result of experimental transmission by injection or by feeding the scrapie agent to these animals.[5] It is relatively easy to keep milk and meat from clinically affected BSE cattle out of the food chain. However, because there are no antemortem (before the cow dies) test to detect infected animals during the protracted incubation stages, our ability to prevent products from cattle, incubating the disease, from entering the food chain is very poor.

## EPIDEMIOLOGICAL INVESTIGATION

Epidemiological investigation strongly suggests that the epidemic was started by feeding cattle protein supplements from sheep meat, and bone meal, which was contaminated by the scrapie agent. When the rendering process was changed in the early 1980s there was a large increase of the incidence of exposure of cattle to the sheep agent of infection (prion). As the disease became established, it may have been amplified by inclusion in rendered products of meat and bone meal from infected cattle. Cattle affected by Mad Cow disease experienced change in temperament, such as nervousness or aggression, loss of body weight despite continued appetite. Finally, they suddenly became very agitated, staggering, snapping and foaming at the mouth before dropping dead.

Hysteria over the mysterious disease was fueled by the death of a Siamese cat named Mac from Bristol which had shown symptoms of BSE where upon the cat was renamed Mad Mac. The cat had been fed pet food made from a beef carcass. At least 70 more cats have died from the spongiform brain lesions (Mad Cat disease), which is associated with the Mad Cow disease. Mad Cow disease has killed more that 161,663 cattle since it was discovered in 1985.

## BOVINE SPONGIFORM ENCEPHALOPATHY

Mad Cow disease has grown to epidemic proportions in the United Kingdom, particularly in the dairy population. The most probable cause was identified as the feeding of sheep scrapie-infected meat and bone meal to cattle. In August of 1988, the slaughter and incineration of BSE cattle was made compulsory. As of November, 1989 a ban on the human consumption of specific bovine offal's (including brain, spinal cord, thymus, spleen, tonsils, and intestines) was imposed. Most recently, a ban on the feeding of all bovine by-products to pet and farm animals was imposed due to the successful experimental transmission of BSE to a pig. Also, since the transmission of BSE to humans is a subject of major concern throughout the United Kingdom and Europe, a study has been initiated to monitor the incidence of human dementia's over the coming years.[6][7][8] The fact that the British government has taken several aggressive steps to control the spread of Mad Cow disease should alert the general public to the health risks involved in the consumption of not only beef, but also dairy products.

## PRIONS

A prion is not a virus or a bacteria. A prion is a protein totally devoid of genetic material, either DNA or RNA. A prion is an agent that cannot be cultured in media or in cell cultures; there is no test to detect the agent (prion) in a live animal; and it does not provoke the development of a specific antibody in the infected animal. Its infectivity still survived a one hour exposure to temperatures as high as 360 degrees Celsius, and auto-claving for 30 minutes at 134 degrees Celsius does not inactivate it. There are few phenomena in the whole of biology that remain totally unaffected by ionizing irradiation, but prions resist irradiation.[9] Prions are what cause the Mad Cow disease in cows. The Mad Cow disease equivalents in humans are the human prion diseases kuru, Gerstmann-Straussler syndrome (GSS), and Creutzfeldt-Jakob disease (CJD) which illustrate three manifestations of central nervous system (brain and spinal cord) degenerative disorders. It has been well documented that all three of these diseases can be transmitted to laboratory animals by inoculation. It can be transmitted to chimpanzees, monkeys and rodents, by injecting their brains with material extracted from the brains of human patients, leads one to believe that they all have a common cause, the prion.

CJD the human equivalent of the Mad Cow disease was epidemic in a small community of Libyan Jews living in Israel is especially interesting, because of having one new case every other month during a several year period. The favorite culprits of transmission have been lightly cooked sheep brain, and other delicacies such as sheep eyeballs, indeed consumption of sheep eyeballs had also been proposed as a mode of transmission. Also, human spongiform encephalopathy, kuru, has reportedly been transmitted between people of primitive societies through ritual cannibalism. The women were predominately affected, this was attributed to the reported custom of women eating the brains and other offal (infected organs), while the men ate the muscle. Presently, the diagnosis of Mad Cow disease is based on observing symptoms and then examining the brain of the deceased cows looking for the holes or rotting of the brain.[10]

## MUTATIONS

There is a potential for direct transmission of BSE to humans. The basic rationale in support of this position assumes that some change or mutation in the scrapie agent permitted it to infect cattle and this modified agent has greater potential to cross other species barriers. Such concern prompted removal of

British beef in May 1990 from the lunch menu from one school district serving 70,000 children. Some other schools, hospitals and retirement homes also removed beef from the menu. The health of various occupational groups such as farmers, packing plant workers, and veterinarians also is being monitored by British officials.

## PRIONS SURVIVAL

In animals, prions are the cause of scrapie in sheep and goats, of transmissible mink encephalopathy, of chronic wasting disease of mule deer and elk, and of BSE in cows. In humans, prions cause kuru, Creutzfeldt-Jakob disease (CJD) and Gerstmann-Straussler syndrome (GSS). The transmissible spongiform encephalopathies can be remembered as Mad Cow disease (BSE); Mad Sheep disease (scrapie); Mad Human disease (CJD); and Mad Mink disease (Transmissible mink encephalopathy TME).

A scrapie-infected hamster brain was mixed with soil, packed into perforated dishes and then mixed with soil in pots and buried in a garden for three years. After three years, the mixture from the soil was still able to cause scrapie, when injected into sheep. This experiment establishes the durability of the scrapie prion exposed to natural environmental conditions for three years, and also shows that most residual infectivity remains in the originally contaminated soil, with little leaching. This explains how in Iceland, healthy flocks of sheep contracted scrapie after being brought to vacant farmland that had three years earlier been grazed by scrapie affected sheep. Because of this it has been suggested that the practice of plowing-under carcasses of animals dying of scrapie or Mad Cow disease, even with the addition of quicklime, be abandoned, and that such animals be excluded as a source of bone meal in fertilizers, unless first autoclaved.

## CAN IT AFFECT HUMANS?

Dr. R.F. Marsh from the University of Wisconsin, a Veterinarian noted for his work on the Mad Cow disease says "You can't dismiss the possibility of the cow disease being transmitted to humans." The United States Department of Agriculture (USDA) stated for years that there was no scientific evidence that indicated that Mad Cow disease is a human health hazard. Now they are changing their minds after the recent outbreak in young teenagers in England. However, concern has been widely voiced by scientists that there was a human health risk. For example Dr. Helen Grant, a neuropathologist formerly at Caring Cross Hospital, says Spongioform Encephalopathy has been passed in the laboratory to chimpanzees. The scientist believe that some mutation in the scrapie agent permitted it to infect cattle, and this modified agent has potential to cross other species barriers.

## MILK FROM MAD COWS

Milk has not yet been proven to transmit Mad Cow disease, and transmission experiments using milk and udder tissue from clinical cases of BSE have, as expected, failed to demonstrate the presence of the agent. Nevertheless, the destruction of milk from suspected cows was recommended by an independent working party chaired by Sir Richard Southwood in England to ensure the public's safety. They also suggested that baby food manufacturers should avoid the use of ruminant brains and other affected organs. Cattle, mice, sheep, goats, and pigs have died in experiments in which the scrapie agent was given by injection or food. Experiments also indicate that temperatures reached during pasteurization of milk and household cooking does not kill the agent. There is no evidence that BSE is transmitted through milk; but there is no conclusive evidence that it can't be. In the United Kingdom on December 1, 1988 the government announced a ban on the sale of milk from infected cattle and that these cattle be destroyed. Unfortunately, animals are infected with the disease long before they show the tell-tale symptoms of the Mad Cow disease and so milk is consumed by humans from cows that are infected with the Mad Cow disease. Just recently the British government has increased the ban on bovine offal's which are prevented from entering the human food chain to include the intestines and thymus of calves under six months old. The action has been taken because of preliminary results from an oral transmission experiment, which indicated that infectivity may develop in the ileum of calves exposed to high doses of the BSE agent more quickly than had been thought. This may be why we still have cows getting the Mad Cow disease in Britain.

## RENDERING

Recently the use of meat and bone meal for calf rations have increased. Currently, the rendering industry sells about 14% of its meat and bone meal to U.S. cattle producers. Most is used as a food protein source for high production dairy cattle and for feed lot cattle.

The USDA has not allowed any federal recommendation against the use of feeding meat and bone meal to young calves, because it feels it would unnecessarily increase the level of concern by consumers and producers. This secretive stance is not well received by the American public; U.S. citizens have come to expect full disclosure.

The recommendations of the USDA are that if BSE is diagnosed in the U.S. decisive steps to stop the use of meat and bone in calf rations should be taken. I say this measure is one that should be enforced right now. At such a point perhaps informed consumers will wonder if this delay was truly necessary. Why can't the U.S. learn from Great Britain's epidemic of BSE and avoid the disaster that occurred to their dairy and beef industry?

## THE BRITISH DISEASE

Why did Mad Cow disease suddenly arrive from nowhere to attack huge numbers of British cattle?[11] [12] In the 1970s rendering businesses switched from and old fashioned technique that used a noxious solvent, and high temperatures, to the American Carver-Greenfield process, which operates at lower temperatures and was meant to make meat and bone meal more nutritious and appetizing. In Britain renderers kept the temperature unusually low, sometimes less than 100 degrees Celsius. A committee of its own experts warned the British government as early as 1980, six years before the first case of BSE, that low temperatures could be dangerous. As soon as other European countries suspected that animal meal might be spreading BSE they prohibited feeding dead cows and sheep to cows and calves. France and Ireland (though not Switzerland) have from the beginning taken the further precaution of destroying all animals in any herd that has seen a case of Mad Cow disease. In July 1988 the British government was prompt to ban the use of cows and sheep to feed to other cows and sheep. This was six months before a government committee, set up to study the problem, gave its report. In August 1988, the British government insisted on the slaughter and destruction of infected animals and of their milk. But the 1988 ban has not been fully enforced. Farmers, who often have a few month's supplies of meal, still had an incentive to get rid of it in the bellies of their cows. Even now, at the back of barns there could be contaminated feed. Worse, with lots of unusable bits of cow and sheep around, feed-makers may have been tempted to smuggle them into food. Nobody knows how much infected material was illegally included in meal. Some believe that offal has continued to be incorporated until recently. That would explain why the BSE epidemic in Britain has still not been brought under control. Though it has peaked, cases are being reported at the rate of over 70 a week. It is also impossible to prevent a few infected animals ending up in slaughterhouses. Even if farmers send no ailing cows to market, some animals may be infectious without showing symptoms of BSE. Abattoirs have been prosecuted for ignoring the rules. Furthermore, even honest slaughterhouses are messy places. Only in November 1995 did the government stop anyone stripping meat from cows' backbones. It had found that small fragments of potentially dangerous spinal cord had been left attached to them, and then the vertebrae had been used in bone meal which contained the agent (prion). Mad Cow disease is not yet out of the human food chain.[13]

## BRAINS OF COWS RIDDLED WITH HOLES

BSE is called a spongiform disease, because the brain becomes riddled with tiny holes giving it the appearance under a microscope of a sponge. Both the human and cow diseases cause sponge-like holes in the brain that gradually disable victims until they die. BSE has a long incubation period. For the disease to manifest itself and eventually kill the cow, it may take from 2 to 8 years.

In the Mad Cow disease, CJD and the other human brain disorders, the infection leads to a slow, lethal degeneration (rotting) of the brain. As noted before prions are extremely resistant to sterilization, indeed formalin fixation of tissues containing the insoluble protein fibrils from the brain (prions) appear to stabilize the agent in surgical specimens. Even after 8 years some of these specimens stored in formalin and then imbedded into paraffin were able to cause the equivalent of the Mad Cow disease in animals. The elapsed time may actually have increased the infectivity.

## MAD COWS AND ENGLISHMEN

Among those who have died in the last three years of Creutzfeldt Jakob Disease (CJD), are four dairy farmers. Some government scientists denied that Bovine Spongiform Encephalopathy popularly called Mad Cow disease could jump to humans and cause CJD, but many other scientists suspect that it does. Now the general public is taking notice of their risks,

Writing in the British Medical Journal, Sheila M. Gore of the government's Medical Research Council suggested that the farmers' deaths "are more than happenstance." Taken with the recently reported deaths of two teenager, they amount to "an epidemiological alert," she said. The scare refuses to go away. For every scientist who says beef is safe, there is one who says it may not be. The scare began in November, 1986 when former government health adviser Sir Bernard Tomlinson, a neuropathologist, said in a radio interview that he had stopped eating hamburgers and products containing beef offal because he fears a link between the human and bovine disease.

Twenty-five percent of the British public now do not eat beef. The number of British vegetarians nearly doubled between 1990 and 1991, from 3.7 percent of the adult population to 7 percent. Vegetarianism is even more popular among 11 to 18 year-olds, with 8 percent describing themselves as vegetarian. At current rates, 28,000 British adults are becoming vegetarian, says the Vegetarian Society of the United Kingdom.[14] On 5/27/96 a poll, done for BBC television, found nearly half of Britain's teen-agers say they have stopped eating beef because of the scare over Mad Cow disease. They also doubted government assurances that the risk of contracting Creutzfeldt-Jakob disease from beef was extremely low.

The public is voting with its fork. According to Nielsen, a research organization in Oxford, 1.4 million households have stopped buying beef. The decline began in November and by mid-December sales were down 25 percent over the same period a year ago. Most affected were hamburgers, with sales at the end of December 1995 down 40 percent. All across the country, schools are taking beef off the menu. Between 5,000 and 7,000 schools have stopped serving it, according to a spokesman for the Local Authority Caterers Association. The British Government banned the use of cow brains in hamburger, a common practice in Britain, and the recycling of sheep in rendering plants.[15]

## MEDICAL PRODUCTS

Food is not the only threat involving the transfer of BSE to humans. Gangliosides represent the active principle of a number of various pharmaceutical products that are actually used in clinics for their neuroregenerative properties. They are found in Health food stores and recommended by Naturopaths for various diseases and symptoms. It is frightening to know that in ganglioside manufacturing procedure it is probably impossible to eliminate completely any possible contamination of prions. Other bovine origin substances that are used in preparation of veterinary or medical products also could be vehicles for spread of the BSE agents, such as Growth hormone, raw pancreas, liver, brains, bone meal and gelatin capsules that contain medicine. Be on the lookout on product labels for ingredients that are usually animal derived unless otherwise indicated: allantoin; amino acids; cholesterol; collagen; elastin; cortisone; fatty acids; glutamic acid; keratin; lipids; nucleic acid; polysorbates; stearic acid, and tallow. There is a lot we as individuals can do to learn more about "hidden" cattle-derived ingredients in common household items, including candies, marshmallows containing gelatin, face cream, and cosmetics.[16]

The opportunities for exposure of man to BSE infection is great because of the use of bovine products in a large range of pharmaceuticals and in food. In monitoring the status of CJD developing in the United Kingdom it would indicate any problem too late to allow preventive action to occur. The thought of having possibly BSE-infected material, used for manufacturing medicine, is fairly horrific, but the situation may worsen. In the U.S., clinical trials are going ahead on the development of a blood substitute for medical use made from purified cow's blood. The association of Medical Microbiologist point out in their excellent leaflet on BSE that BSE-type agents show amazing resistance to heat, chemical agents and irradiation and are not completely killed by boiling, or immersion for years in formalin. The production of parenteral animal drugs and material infected with scrapie/BSE agent may increase the risk of disease transmission. The majority of these products would be USDA regulated biologicals. However, some hormones, and drugs such as insulin and heparin, produced from bovine source material and regulated would also pose a risk if contaminated with BSE when used in susceptible animals and humans. It has been recommended that producers of human and animal drugs and biologics not use source material from BSE positive countries. But no law has been enacted. It is only suggested that they not be used.

## PITUITARY HORMONE THERAPY

There are 23 known cases of CJD attributable to treatment with human growth hormone obtained from pituitaries of human cadavers This hormone was given to dwarfs and children who appeared not to be growing to their normal height. At least six more cases are suspected in France. These individuals unfortunately, remain at risk for several decades to come, because incubation periods may be as long as 35 years. The introduction of purification procedures in 1977 did not, as hoped, achieve total decontamination of the hormone extracts. The human pituitary hormones were replaced by synthetic preparations in 1985, but a few countries inexplicably continue to use hormones from the pituitary glands from dead humans. This practice should cease. Regrettably the medical profession has caused CJD resulting from various types of therapeutic interventions. It is a serious and growing problem in the high-technology of modern medicine.[17]

## INSPECTING COW BRAINS

From 1986, to March 21, 1996, U.S. diagnosticians at the National Veterinary Services Laboratories inspected 2,791 bovine brains for signs of bovine spongiform encephalopathy (BSE). None were positive. This is a tiny fraction of the total population of 103 million cattle, and is totally inadequate. BSE which has an incubation period of up to eight years, may not be detectable in American beef cattle, many of which are slaughtered between the ages of two and five.

In the United Kingdom as of August 1991, there had been more than 40,000 infected cattle with about 500 new cases being discovered each week.[18] Then in 1992 and 1993 new cases in Great Britain approached a staggering figure of 10,000 monthly. The good news was that more recently, between September 1 and December 1, 1995, Great Britain reported only 3,151 newly confirmed cases of BSE with 272 more herds affected. This is a welcomed decline. It is felt that this decline was due to the fact that it was against the law to feed sheep and cows to cows. But the ban was not completely followed so the epidemic continues. As of December 1, 1995, the total number of confirmed cases equaled 155,621; total number of affected herds stood at 32,991; 54.1 percent of the dairy herds have been affected.

## MAD MINK DISEASE

Transmissible mink encephalopathy (TME) or Mad Mink disease is food borne disease of ranch-raised mink. It is produced by an unidentified contaminated feed ingredient. It was initially assumed that TME was caused by feeding mink scrapie-infected sheep. However, subsequent studies testing the oral susceptibility of mink to scrapie were unsuccessful, but now there have occurred two incidents in which the mink rancher was confident that sheep were not fed to his animals. The most recent of these was in Stetsonville, Wisconsin in 1985 where the meat portion of the diet was composed of almost exclusively downer dairy cows. Anyone who eats beef in America should be reminded of this epidemic. Beef caused the Mad Mink disease in the United States. So it is possible that beef can do a similar thing in the human United States population.

As the consequences of the above information we must examine the outbreak of the mad mink disease more closely. In April 1985, the owner of a mink ranch in Stetsonville, Wis., called the Ranch Service to report that many of his animals were behaving abnormally and that some had died. Upon visiting the ranch it was apparent that approximately 400 animals were showing various clinical stages of TME (Mad Mind disease). The earliest signs were behavioral changes, in which the mink appeared to be hyperexcitable and no longer deposited feces in a single area of the pen but distributed fecal material randomly throughout the cage. Arching of the tail over the back in a squirrel-like manner was observed in many animals. Mink at more advanced stages showed a lack of locomotor coordination, as evidenced by their inability to climb into their nestboxes or to maintain their hindquarters in a straight standing position when at rest. Some mink appeared completely somnolent with their noses in the corner of the cage as if in a trance. The length of clinical illness until death varied from two weeks in some mink to six weeks in others.

The disease persisted on the ranch for five months. Of the total breeding herd of 7,300 adult animals, approximately 60% developed clinical signs, and all of these died. The ranch owner stated that most of the fresh meat portion of the minks diet had come from fallen and sick dairy cattle which were picked up within a fifty mile radius of the mink ranch and returned for processing (butchering, grinding and freezing). A few horses had also been used. Sheep products were never fed to the mink and there were no feed supplements of meat and bone meal. These events suggest there are no species barriers between mink and cattle for the Mad Cow disease and the Mad Mink disease. It also shows that the prion can cross the species barrier. Remember our cows are fed scrapie (Mad Sheep disease) infected sheep which is widespread in the United States and thousands of dead downer cows that may be infected with prions.

Supporting this is Dr. R.F. Marsh from the University of Wisconsin, a noted specialist on scrapie (Mad Sheep disease) and the Mad Cow disease, is one of those who believes it is possible that there exists as yet an undetected source of sheep scrapie capable of producing disease in mink after ingestion of downer cows. His conclusion is based on the following experiment.

Two Holstein steers each developed Mad Cow disease 18 and 19 months after being inoculated with Stetsonville infected portions of the mad mink brains.[19] The brain tissue from these two Holstein steers that died of the Mad Cow disease were fed to well mink and these mink developed in only seven months the Mad Mink disease (TME). These findings are compatible with the suggestion that the Stetsonville incident of Mad Mink disease was produced by feeding an infected "downer cow" to mink. March's conclusions are there must exist a previously unrecognized Mad Cow disease (BSE)-like infection in American cattle. The U.S. version of Mad Cow disease, however, did not produce the behavioral symptoms--staggering and drooling--that made the disease obvious in British cattle. Instead, the two steers experimentally infected by Marsh died by simply collapsing, mimicking a common cow ailment in the U.S. called

"Downer Cow Syndrome." Over 20,000 "downer" cows die each year in Wisconsin alone. A U.S. BSE agent could be hidden in this large population. Downer cows are typically rendered and fed back to living cows, which could concentrate and amplify the disease into an epidemic like the one that has devastated the British cattle industry, but harder to detect because the cows would not go "mad" before keeling over dead. A major U.S. outbreak seems plausible, even likely, unless the U.S. government acts swiftly to outlaw the practice of feeding rendered byproduct protein (ruminants) to cows.

"We are in a mass experiment which is killing us," says Tim Lang, professor of Food Policy at Thames Valley University. "Never before have diseased ruminants (sheep) been fed to other ruminants (cows) and then fed to humans. We have interfered with the whole process of nature and what is now happening is one of our worst nightmares. This is a tragedy on a massive scale. The Government has been so totally stupid. Even now they are still employing crisis management techniques and damage limitation exercises."

"It now appears I was wrong," admits U.S. medical official Dr. Paul Brown. "A great deal of work remains to be done. . . Nor will it remedy the possible failure of the scientific pundits (including me) to foresee a potential medical catastrophe."[20] When the Health Ministry announced the latest in a series of CJD deaths that are so different from the textbook description of the disease--the victims were young, the brain tissue looked like Alzheimer's--that they suggest a link to Mad Cows, says Dr. Paul Brown of the U.S. National Institutes of Health. Dr. Brown, a leading Creutzfeldt-Jakob disease researcher with the National Institutes of Health, believes that humans may be able to contract CJD from infected cattle parts even if they don't eat them. Theoretically, just applying a moisturizer that contain collagen from a "Mad Cow" could expose the user to CJD. There is no hard evidence that CJD has been transmitted this way. But if by-products do turn out to be source of infection the potential for disaster is mind-boggling. They're used in everything from shampoo to floor wax. The USDA says it doesn't keep track of how much beef by-product is imported from England and other countries where mad cow disease has been detected.[21]

What is the origin of TME (Mad Mink disease)? If the disease results from feeding infected cattle to mink, what is its relationship to BSE (Mad Cow disease) and why did we not identify a BSE-like disease in American cattle? One possible explanation is that this rare disease of cattle has not had an opportunity to be transmitted in the United States. Contrary to Great Britain, animal protein has only been used extensively in American cattle feed for the past 10-12 years. Currently we are feeding a minimum of 14% of all rendered cattle back to other cattle. This practice certainly increases the possibility for transmission of a Mad Cow disease BSE-like agent. Certainly there is reason for concern because the danger of this trend is magnified when the American cattle industry is using more meat and bone meal in cattle rations than any other countries. Furthermore these neuropathological agents (prions) are very likely to survive any conventional rendering process of the meat and bones. Cows trust man, but man has become their worst nightmare. Animal husbandry have boosted a single cows milk production from the traditional 20 pounds of milk a day to today's average of more than three times that much. Cows have become our primary recycling agents in our society. We feed cows orange skins, almond husks, dead sheep, and chicken manure. Yes, cows eat dead sheep and cows. That leads up to unconscious cow cannibalism. And did you ever wonder about what happens to all those feathers plucked from the chickens and turkeys we eat. They are ground up and mixed with the dead sheep and cows and become cow food. The cows don't know what they are eating or they would really get mad. It is sold to the dairyman as a Dairy Supplement that contains a special bypass protein called PNP, Protected Natural Protein to get more milk from the dairy cows. Many dairyman do not know what they are feeding their cows either.

Finally, we should not expect that a BSE-like disease in the United States would necessarily have to have all of the features of BSE (Mad Cow disease) in Great Britain. The existence of distinct biologic strains of these transmissible agents is well documented. The cattle inoculated with the Stetsonville mink brain showed no behavioral changes before collapsing in their pens. What if the strain of BSE (Mad Cow disease) in American cattle produces more of a "downer cow syndrome" than "Mad Cow syndrome" and is a different mutated strain of the Mad Cow disease? This eventually would definitely complicate surveillance programs for BSE in the United States. Our country has hundreds of thousands of downer cows each year and no means for routinely diagnosing their cause.[22] [23]

## SCIENTIST GIVE UP BEEF

In reviewing the information about Mad Cow disease, I have reached the conclusion that at this time beef products should be avoided. This conclusion has been validated by many in the scientific community of Great Britain. The advice of Professor Richard Lacey of Leeds University is: "The only logical approach for the human population in the United Kingdom is to avoid all beef products."

The Rowett Research Institute in Scotland is a world leader in animal and food-related research. Its animal and food research has won it great respect in the scientific community but it's findings will win it few friends in the cattle industry. It came as a quite a shock to the establishment, when Rowett Director, Prof. Philip Hames declared, at the Oxford Farming Conference, in January of 1991, that he had given up eating beef three years before the BSE scare, as he had had advance notice about the disease.

The seriousness of the situation is underlined by the following statement. A Leeds University Medical School colleague of Prof. Lacey's, Dr. Stephen Dealler, says that if humans eat infected meat they will have a 50/50 chance of getting the disease. He concludes "No one who knows enough about this subject would feed their daughter a beef burger."[24] He stated in the British Food Journal that most adult British meat-eaters will by 2001, have ingested a potentially fatal dose of meat infected with BSE. It seems that those closely involved in researching BSE are impressed enough to change their lifestyles.

## USDA STAND ON RENDERED CARCASSES OF SHEEP

In early December of 1989, the U.S. National Renderers Association (NRA) sent a letter to renderers requesting that they refuse to pick up dead, dying, diseased, or disabled sheep and that they divert all protein produced from sheep offal to feed use other than cattle feeds. In response to this Carl Osborn, Department of Veterinary Medicine (DVM) in a briefing letter on BSE stated that it is the departments position that the action taken by the US National Renderers Association is unjustified at this time. In a memorandum of telephone conversation to a feed company executive George Graber, Ph.D. Director, Division of Animal Feeds, USDA pointed out that the National Renders Association was the principle driving force behind the request not to render sheep. The directive/recommendation to ban ruminant offal in rendered products is not an FDA document. After noting all of the above information, it is hard to believe that any knowledgeable person in authority could deny that some action should be taken, however, John Honstead DVM on July 24, 1991 said that FDA should not, at that time, recommend a ban on ruminant offal in rendered products destined for cattle feeding.

In 1989 the stand of the U.S. National Renderers Association (NRA) was right and the FDA was wrong. The NRA apparently was discouraged after the FDA and USDA disapproval of a voluntary band of feeding ruminants to ruminants. It was never carried out as reported by the FDA in the Federal Register of 1993. The philosophy the FDA and the USDA in making decisions is that if you can't prove something scientifically then it must not be right. They argue that nothing has been proven yet. They ignore the Delaney amendment and common sense. They believe if it has not been published in the scientific journals, then it has not been proven yet. Because of this reasoning thousands of people will die horrible deaths. In the 1980's how could we prove that feeding dead cows and sheep that had cancer, infectious diseases would result in the Mad Cow disease. But by using our intelligence we could have prevented it. This is what happened in Britain with the Mad Cow epidemic. We can only wait and see how many people die of CJD because of this type of decision making. Here in the United States we can play Russian roulette and continue to feed our cows infected cows and sheep that have cancer and infectious disease organism or we can follow the Precautionary Principle of Preventive Medicine of being safe rather than sorry. We can base our decisions on epidemiological, statistical data when scientific evidence actually is still inconclusive. An example of this reasoning is the astonishing statement that was a bit of information on the Mad Cow disease in a CDC memorandum advising state epidemiologists that there is no evidence of human health risk at this time. As pointed out in this chapter we have already seen that many scientists disagree with this assessment. Another example of this is Lung cancer and cigarette smoking. In a later chapter on Retroviruses I will discuss scientific evidence more fully.

Briefing information on BSE by Carl G. Osborne, DVM July 26, 1990 revealed the astonishing fact that total U.S. production of rendered products in 1989 was 5.5 million metric tons (12.1 billion lb.). Think how many diseased dead cows that represents and the amazing potential for the transfer of diseases to livestock and humans. We know that infectious diseases in animals and humans are increasing in epidemic proportions. As a Preventive Medicine and Public Health epidemiologist I am concerned. Infectious disease specialists, and the CDC are alarmed. We can stop this rising epidemic by discontinuing feeding cancerous, diseased animals to animals that are used as food for humans.

## DEAD COWS FED TO COWS TO PRODUCE MORE MILK

Cows are being fed dead cows in order to make them produce more milk. The meat, bones, blood meal, and soybean is mixed up into pellets, and fed to cows to make them 'super cows'. It is sold in feed mixtures as "undegradable bypass protein." It is advertised in dairy magazines such as Hoards Dairyman in colorful pictures of dairy life in full page adds.

Most dairyman do not know what is in the mixture. All they know is that it increases the cows milk production.[25]

Professor RF Marsh from the University of Wisconsin and international authority on Mad Cow disease believes that the US should stop the widespread practice of feeding its cattle feed mixtures containing cattle protein, because of the risks of an outbreak of the Mad Cow disease. Britain has already had to introduce such a ban because of BSE. "If we don't stop feeding our cattle this animal protein we're setting ourselves up for the same thing as happened in Britain." He said. The main lesson to be learned is that animals should be fed food appropriate to their species. Common sense tells us it was a bad idea to feed animal wastes to herbivorous creatures, especially cows that end up on our dinner tables![26]

## MISDIAGNOSED DEMENTIA CASES

Some doctors have suggested that patients currently being treated for mental illness may in fact have Creutzfeldt-Jacobs Disease. Evidence given by F.G. Roberts suggests that the true figure for the number of humans who die from this type of disease (CJD) every year in the UK should be revised from around thirty upwards to a possible 9,000! Of the 75,000 people who die demented, he believes around two percent have a disease of this type but that many of them never have a definite diagnosis.[27]

It may not be only in Britain, however, where causes of dementia are misdiagnose. In order to study the accuracy of clinicians in predicting the pathologic diagnosis the Departments of Neurology of the Veterans Administration Medical Center, and the University of Pittsburgh Medical School, Pittsburgh, Pa. Autopsied 54 demented patients. Two neurologists independently reviewed the clinical records of each patient; 20% were incorrect in the diagnosis. These results show that in patients with a clinical diagnosis of dementia, the etiology cannot be accurately predicted during life.[28] In the United States, death or severe disability due to Alzheimer's disease is a major hazard. Today, 4 million Americans have Alzheimer's disease or a related disorder. By the year 2050 14 million Americans will have Alzheimer's unless medical science finds a way to prevent or halt the progress of the disease. One in 10 persons over age 65, and nearly half of those over age 85, have probable Alzheimer's. One in three American families is affected by Alzheimer's disease. Alzheimer's disease costs the nation over $90 billion a year. Families pay virtually all of that cost. Considering the information that is accumulating, one can not help but wonder how many of those 20% missed diagnosis are related to CJD. Interestingly enough an editorial in the Lancet, the highly respected British medical journal (7/7/90) suggests that prion disease in humans is often mis-diagnosed and that, whereas official figures for Creutzfeldt-Jakob disease run at 30-40 cases per year in the United Kingdom, a more realistic figure would be 4,500!

On 3/23/89, neurologist Drs. Helen Grant and William Blackwood of Charing Cross and Westminister Medical School published a letter in The Times that pointed out that unless bovine brain is totally banned from human food or is avoided, a new human health hazard hovers over us; the risk of an untreatable dementia. It looks like their prophecy is coming true. Further support for their belief comes from prion research which has major implications for understanding many common brain disorders. According to Dr. Donald Price, a prominent brain researcher at the John Hopkins Medical School in Baltimore, a similar kind of protein abnormality might underlie the changes seen in the brains of Alzheimer's and Parkinson's patients. [29]

## DOCTORS WARN OF BSE TIME BOMB

Neurologist, D. R. Robert, at the Western General Hospital, Edinburgh, who has a government grant to monitor the human equivalent of BSE, Creutzfeldt-Jakob disease said the issue 'will be a question for another 15 years if Mad Cow disease is a threat to human health.' While scientific certainty may still be 15 years away, there is enough evidence for individuals such as those researchers I mentioned earlier to protect ourselves. If our children and grandchildren are going to be protected from this horrible disease there is enough information for us to do the right thing now. A stitch in time saves nine and strike while the iron is hot is applicable today. I believe the American public is health conscious and will turn America around by standing up for what they know is right by not eating beef until changes are made. There is enough evidence for us to make this decision. It is the only way that the Beef and Dairy industries will be persuaded to stop feeding dead cows and sheep to cows.

## MAD COW JUMPS THE SPECIES BARRIER AGAIN

Three ostriches from German zoos have developed a brain disease similar to the Mad Cow disease. Their brains showed the spongy holes typical of the brains from cattle infected with the Mad Cow disease. The ostriches had been fed some raw meat from a local "emergency slaughter" abattoir. German researchers claim that in spite of this apparent transmission to ostriches, commercially reared poultry should not pose a danger to human health because they are slaughtered and eaten so early in life before the brain disease could develop in chickens and turkeys.[30] In other words, they seem to believe that it is safe to eat a disease bearing hosts simply because the hosts has no symptoms yet! This is a difficult logic to accept.

## SCRAPIE IN THE UNITED STATES

As I discussed earlier the spongform disease in sheep is called Scrapie (mad sheep disease) because those that are infected tend to scrape themselves against fences, rocks, and walls. It is a brain disorder which is believed to affect animals, but rarely, humans. Scrapie in the United States was first introduced by Suffolk sheep imported from Britain, and was first reported in 1947 in Michigan. A voluntary scrapie eradication program began in 1952. Since 1979, however the number of flocks in which scrapie has been diagnosed has increased greatly. From 1984 through 1988 the numbers reported were nearly three times the number during any previous years. In one flock of Suffolk sheep in Iowa, 50 percent of lambs born in

1986 died to the disease. Geographically in the United States, it has been reported in all but 11 states.[31] According to the USDA, about 7,500 American sheep have the disease. The USDA says there is no evidence that scrapie prion has caused disease in humans. The occurrence of scrapie in the U.S. has limited the export of breeding stock because other countries do not want to have scrapie in their country. The USDA believes there is no evidence that scrapie can be transmitted to man but it appears to be perceived to be a potential public health threat by some and that it is implied by the existing control programs to eliminate scrapie in the United States. So the USDA discontinued the compulsory eradication program because it would be perceived by the public that it was a threat to health. Any methods for control or elimination of Scrapie by the U.S. government has now been given up. Is this just typical government double think, or is it a deliberate attempt to keep the truth from the public? Certainly there is enough evidence for us to ask, "why are we feeding scrapie infected sheep to our dairy cows in the United States?" Doing so simply defies common sense. Although there is no evidence that scrapie can be transmitted directly to man it is clearly perceived to be a potential public health threat by many as is implied by the existence of foreign and domestic control programs. I believe the higher rate of scrapie in sheep in the United States pose an increasing threat to humans. In contrast to the sheep situation, very few cases of scrapie have been diagnosed in goats in the United States, and the diligence of careful goat owners can help keep the incidence of scrapie in goats low.

So the USDA discontinued the compulsory eradication program, because it would be perceived by the public that it was a threat to health!

**NOVEL**

A novel "Sacred Cow" published in Omni magazine January 1993 depicted the conditions fifty years after the Mad Cow epidemic. The novel describes over one million people being buried in one mass grave in England. The living, fearing a plague, shipped the dead out of London in a train to be buried. In this fictional projections of the future every sheep and cow that might have any infection was killed in order to wipe out scrapie, then it was supposedly perfectly safe to eat beef. Ninety percent of Britain, thirty percent of Western Europe, twenty percent of America, dead because of hamburgers. [32] This, of course, is fiction, but it may still provide a warning and we can prevent it from happening.

## RECENT EVENTS

New York Times front page, Thursday, March 21, 1996 screamed "Britain Ties Deadly Brain Disease to Cow Ailment"! Robert Lacey, professor of microbiology at Leeds University, warned the public of a possible link between Mad Cow disease in cows and the human disease Creutzfeldt-Jakob Disease. These two diseases, even thought they are in different mammals, have the same symptoms-and both lead to death! Lacey informed the British government long ago that Mad Cow disease, could be traced to the disease of scrapie in sheep. He believes that scrapie somehow crossed the species barrier into cows through the practice of feeding cows bone and meat remnants including brains, from sheep. These sheep remains are routinely ground up and fed to cows as a protein supplement. Lacey warns, that there is a seventy percent chance it will move on to another species. Most likely the next species will be humans, as we are seeing signs of the beginning of a human epidemic. This is one of the most disgraceful episodes in this country's history. The reason action was not taken is that it would be expensive and damaging politically, particularly to the farming community who are their supporters. The deadly cover-up Lacey deplored in England is continuing today in the United States. Unfortunately, internal documents and plans obtained by PR Watch, editor John Stauber, investigations show that the government has sought to protect the economic interests of the powerful meat and animal feed industries, while denying the existence of risks to animals and humans.

Britain's Health Secretary, Stephen Dorrell, told the House of Commons on March 21, 1996, that a committee of scientists had linked an unusual outbreak of the human disease, Creutzfeldt-Jakob Disease, to exposure to cows infected with the Mad Cow disease! Exposure to Mad Cow disease through the consumption of beef years ago is the most likely reason why an apparently new variant of the deadly brain disease is surfacing today in young people.

Scientists in Great Britain have reported that ten people under the age of forty-two, some only in their teens, have Creutzfeldt-Jakob Disease. Eight of these ten people have died and the other two are seriously ill. This rare disease normally only affects the middle aged and elderly. Creutzfeldt-Jakob Disease is increasing in Great Britain. This disease usually affects only one in a million people, but has nearly doubled between 1990 and 1994.

The British government has been embarrassed by its about-face on its stand regarding the safety of British beef. The government now states for the first time that there very well may be a link between the Mad Cow disease in cows and the dreadful and deadly neurological disease in humans. When concern first arose in 1990, the British government adamantly insisted that there was no link between the two diseases, or that, in case one were established, preventative procedures were in place to keep the parts of cattle likely to cause infection out of the human food chain. In the early 1990's British Agriculture Minister, John Gummer, went on television with his four year old daughter and fed her a hamburger made from British cows to demonstrate that British beef was perfectly safe! It now appears that it was not safe for human consumption. Wisely, schools in Great Britain immediately dropped beef from lunch menus, because of the fear of Mad Cow disease. The out cry against the British beef industry has been so great that the Prime Minister of Britain, John Majors, has had to address the Mad

38

Cow issue and it has taken up much of his time as Prime Minister. One hopes that this is not a case where fact follows fiction as depicted in the novel, Sacred Cow.

Since BSE emerged scientists and consumers have been haunted by the thought that it could be transmitted to humans. The human equivalent to BSE is Creutzfeldt-Jakob Disease, which mainly affects the elderly and causes loss of memory, grinding headaches, tripping and stumbling as the nerves of the victims legs give out. As the rotting of the brain continues all muscles go slack and flabby, with loss of coordination and a lethal psychotic stupor sets in with blindness and eventually death.

Up to 1.4 million households in Britain stopped buying beef by December 1995, according to a market research team in Britain because of fear of contracting the Mad Cow disease. Fears that the disease could jump the barrier between cattle and humans and cause a similar fatal brain disease in people were exacerbated when several leading scientists said they had stopped eating burgers and pies made with beef.

In December of 1995 hundreds of schools took beef off their menus after pressure from concerned parents and Meat sales fell by 25 percent. In February 1996 it was reported by a scientist that the human form of the Mad Cow disease had claimed the life of a 20-year-old man. In February 1996, Bavaria, North Rhine-Westphalia and Rhineland-Palatinate, in Germany banned imports of British beef to ease consumers' fears they could be infected with the Mad Cow disease. Many of Germany's 16 federal states say Britain has failed to eradicate the disease from its cattle, and that there is no proof that the Mad Cow disease cannot be transmitted to humans.

## ECONOMIC CONCERNS

The British government has put economic concerns above human health for too long. Now it is no longer just a British concern, but a world health problem, and the United States is following in the footsteps of Britain's mistakes. In the United States as well, it appears that economic concerns are being put above health concerns.

Mad Cow disease has caused an enormous stampede against British beef. France, Belgium and Sweden banned imports of British immediately after Health Secretary Dorrell's announcement. To prevent any possible spread of the incurable disease, Germany called for a ban on British beef in the European Community. Top British health officials indicate that it will probably be necessary to slaughter all of Britain's eleven million cattle to stop the deadly brain disease in its tracks! Financial experts estimate the cost of the slaughter could cost the British government 30.76 billion.

Unfortunately the United States did not ban British beef imports until 1989, three years after the Mad Cow disease was first diagnosed in 1986. Veterinarians with the USDA's Animal and Plant Health Inspection Service are in the process of tracking down 499 head of cattle imported from Great Britain between 1981 and 1989 to check their health status. The USDA said as of January 22, 1996 in the United States, 106 British cattle are known to be alive, 341 cattle are known to be dead and eight of the British imported cattle have been exported. Linda Detwiler, DVM a veterinary scientist with the USDA says of the cattle that died may have been sent to slaughterhouses for rendering. "Theoretically, tainted British beef could have infected American cattle." The USDA says it cannot account for 35 of the cows. According to the United States government there are no known cases of Mad Cow disease in the United States. However, don't be fooled the Mad Cow is the consumers enemy all over the world.

## SUMMARY

For seven years the U.S. Department of Agriculture (USDA), the Food and Drug Administration (FDA), and the multi-billion dollar animal livestock industry have cooperated in a cover-up of huge health risks to animals and people in the United States. For 10 years, even preceding the British outbreak of Mad Cow Disease, the USDA has had scientific evidence that a version of the disease exists in U.S. cattle. Yet government and industry have failed even at this late date to ban the practice of "cow cannibalism" which created the fatal epidemic now spreading in Britain from cows to people. The practice has been banned in Britain for years, but continues in the U.S. and is in fact more widespread here than in any other country. The feeding of ruminant protein (sheep and cows) to cows continues at a rate of millions of pounds per day. [33]

Recent studies conducted with macaque monkeys provide the strongest evidence yet that the human form of mad cow disease may possibly come from cattle. Dr. Adriano Aguzzi, chief of the National Survey Program for Creutzfeldt-Jakob Disease in Switzerland commented: "In my view it ends the debate that it didn't come from cows. On the one hand, now we can say this is something that can happen...the disease coming up in the monkeys is identical to the human disease found in Great Britain."

The monkeys tested developed mad cow disease three years after having been injected with brain tissue from British cows. The macaque monkeys developed unmistakable symptoms of the mad cow disease. Aguzzi expressed marked concern because rationed amount of the infectious disease infected was "well-within the range of brain tissue present in commercial food products for human consumption until a few years ago". Aguzzi cited that the disease "shows a characteristic never seen before...it is highly promiscuous in its choice of hosts. Unlike its counterpart in sheep mice and hamsters, it appears to infect animals of other species easily, especially when transmitted orally." Aguzzi called for research to be conducted with the macaque ingesting the brain tissue instead of having it injected.

41

The Journal of the American Medical Association reporting from the results of the World Health Organization recommendation of April 2-3, 1996, based on the latest scientific information, to minimize transmission of BSE among animals and to reduce as completely as possible any exposure of humans to the BSE agent. (1) Countries should not permit tissues that are likely to contain the BSE agent to enter any food chain, human or animal. (2) All countries should ban the use of ruminant tissues in ruminant feed.[34] In spite of this recommendation we continue to feed our cows dead cows and sheep. The FDA refuses to believe this is a emergency. It may be a whole year before the FDA will stop this horrible practice. Is the FDA dragging its feet in order for the dairyman renderers and beef producers to use up the feed they now have in their barns? How stupid can we be?

Mad Cow disease (BSE) has raised questions concerning feeding practices in Agriculture, food safety, the speed at which government responds to new epidemics, and general government competence and commitment to human safety. We are ultimately led to the 'bottom-line question', 'when are we going to cease this despicable practice?" We can't allow this to happen any more in America.

# CHAPTER TWO

# PETITION TO FDA

On June 16, 1993, The Foundation on Economic Trends, and its president, Jeremy Rifkin filed a petition requesting the Food and Drug Administration (FDA) to halt the feeding of ruminant animal protein to ruminants. I was the medical consultant for the Petition. In the petition we requested the FDA and the USDA take the following action to prevent the potential spread of a severe health threat to both animals and humans: 1)order a permanent halt to all feeding of ruminant animal protein to ruminants, especially cows and sheep; 2) develop a significant epidemiological investigation to determine the incidence of transmissible spongiform encephalopathies (TSE), such as scrapie-like diseases in sheep (Mad Sheep Disease) and bovine spongiform encephalopathy-like (Mad Cow Disease) diseases in cattle, among ruminant animals in the United States: (ruminant animals chew the cud); 3) develop a separate, significant epidemiological study to determine the incidences of (TSE) in "downer" cattle (cows that can't stand, because they are so sick, or have died, and are fed back to the cows for increased milk production); 4) establish a bovine brain bank for the ongoing study of TSE's; 5) develop a significant epidemiological investigation to determine the incidence of transmissible spongiform encephalopathies among the human population of the United States; and 6) develop an ongoing national monitoring and registry program utilizing autopsy examinations to determine any changes in the incidence  CJD-like diseases among the human population of the United States.

The petition was 10 pages long and I will now just include some of the highlights of the petition. John Stauber  worked extensively in developing the petition and I provided medical advise to help him in it's preparation.

**STATEMENT OF FACTS**

43

The health and safety of ruminant animals, primarily cows and sheep, are at grave risk because of the relatively recent and increasing practice of feeding ruminant animal protein—the otherwise unmarketable remains of rendered cows and sheep—to cows and other ruminants in the form of commercial animal feed products.

Currently, end products from rendering are being used to feed ruminant animals throughout the United States. The rendering industry utilizes packing house offal, meat processing waste, restaurant waste and animal tissues from other sources including animals that have died otherwise than by slaughter.[35]

Sheep in the U.S. have been infected for at least forty years with the disease scrapie (Mad Sheep Disease), a transmissible spongiform encephalopathy (TSE) which survives the rendering process and can be transmitted to animals that consume feed made in part from the infected remains of these ruminant animals. There is evidence that a TSE-like agent also currently infects an unknown number of cows in the U.S. In 1985 an outbreak of transmissible mink encephalopathy(TME, Mad Mink Disease) was discovered at a mink ranch in Wisconsin. The mink's diet consisted of 95% "downer cows" and 5% horse meat.[36] The mink consumed no sheep meat so the scrapie agent has been ruled out as a source of the TME outbreak.

Subsequent studies have shown that when cows are injected with either the TME or scrapie agents, the animals exhibit characteristics of "downer" cow syndrome and die from a TSE-like disease.[37]

As a result, researchers have concluded that the "downer" cows may have been the source of the Wisconsin minks' infectious TSE agent. If this is the case, thousands of "downer" cattle in the U.S. may be the result of a previously unrecognized TSE-like agent in cattle. In Europe a TSE agent, commonly referred to as Bovine Spongiform Encephalopathy (BSE) or "Mad Cow Disease." Has been implicated in the death of numerous cattle.

In the U.S. virtually every "downer" cow is sent to a slaughterhouse where they are readied for human consumption and/or made into high protein animal feed. This feeding of slaughtered cows (especially "downer cows") and sheep to healthy cow and sheep herds risks the concentration and spread of scrapie and TSE-like agents among ruminants. Moreover, the ability of TSE agents to cross species lines through the consumption of infected protein raises a severe concern about a possible "zoonotic" effect in humans as a result of consuming contaminated beef. (Zoonosis is a scientific term for any disease which originates in animals and can be passed on to humans sometimes in a much more virulent form.).

Transmissible spongiform encephalopathies occur in many species, including humans, and can be transmitted by consumption of infected materials. In humans TSE is most commonly referred to as Creutzfeldt-Jacob Disease (CJD). There is a long latency period of 10 to 30 years between human exposure to a TSE agent and the appearance of dementia symptoms, after which CJD is 100% fatal in humans within 1 year of the appearance of dementia symptoms.

As a result of CJD close physical relationship to TSE's there is a significant concern that the consumption of TSE-infected cattle or sheep, or cattle and sheep fed TSE-infected ruminant protein, could have a direct impact on human health by promoting the onset of CJD. In fact, there already are several indications that incidences of CJD in the United States are on the rise. There is much overlap in symptomatology between Alzheimer's Disease (AD) and CJD. Studies indicate a typical 25% error rate in the clinical diagnosis of dementia.[38] Up to 4 million Americans currently are thought to be afflicted with Alzheimer's Disease, the leading dementia disease. The specific causes of AD are unknown at this time, but hypotheses include head trauma, prion infectious, aluminum toxicity, and immunologic disorders.

If an increasing number of people are developing CJD, their deaths could be hidden by the high number of Alzheimer's cases, since direct post-mortem evaluation of brain tissue is the only positive method of determining whether a patient has Alzheimer's Disease or CJD. Researchers have recommended that direct neuropathological examination at autopsy be undertaken in all demented patients to determine the actual incidence of the various dementia diseases, including CJD, but only a small number of dementia victims are now autopsied.

Often CJD is confused with other forms of dementia. When doctors at the Veterans Administration Medical Center in Pittsburgh, Pennsylvania, consecutively autopsied 54 demented patients, they discovered that three (5.5%) had died of CJD disease, a rate of CJD occurrence that is about one thousand times higher than expected.[39]

Despite these indications that TSE agents and CJD pose a serious potential health risk to both the nation's cattle herds and meat-eating consumers, the FDA and USDA has yet to ban a potential source of TSE spread, the practice of feeding ruminant animal protein to ruminants, or to undertake a significant epidemiological study to determine the prevalence of TSE-like diseases among cattle or CJD among humans.

### STATEMENT OF THE LAW

Food and Drug Administration, Compliance Policy Guide 7126.24 (10-1-80) states: Rendered animal feed ingredients which contain harmful microorganisms, toxins or chemical substances may be considered adulterated under Sections 402(a)(1) or (2) of the Act. Where a rendering procedure itself raises a question of disease transmission, the ingredient made may be deemed adulterated under Section 402(a)(4).[40]

### ARGUMENT

The general delegation of power to FDA and USDA to take the actions requested herein is found generally at 21 U.S.C. Section 371, et seq. and 21 U.S.C. Section 111 respectively. In addition, the FDA is "lead" agency in deciding matters under the auspices of the Federal Food, Drug and Cosmetic Act (FFDCA). The Secretary of Agriculture's opinion regarding the usefulness of feeding ruminant animal protein to ruminants is only one of the many factors which the FDA must consider in responding to this petition.[41]

A. The FDA should immediately halt all feeding of ruminant animal protein to ruminants, especially sheep and cows.

Sheep in the U.S. have been infected for at least forty years with the disease scrapie, a transmissible spongiform encephalopathy (TSE) which survives the rendering process and can be transmitted to cows and sheep that consume feed composed of the infected remains of ruminant animals. It has been increasingly recognized that TSE's can be transmitted across species lines through direct injection of the disease into an animal or through the ingestion of infected animal protein by an animal. For example, researchers have found the scrapie TSE to have survived in calves after a direct clinical application.[42] In addition, several clinical research experiments have documented the transferability of a TSE from cattle to mink as a result of the minks' ingestion of infected cattle feed.[43]

On a national average approximately fourteen percent of all cattle by mass are fed back to cattle in the form of rendered animal protein. The prevalence of rendered animal protein in animal diets is significantly higher in states with large bovine populations. Similarly, a recent Center for Veterinary Medicine survey of rendering plants found that 25% of plants surveyed were still rendering sheep for use by cattle feed producers despite the National Renderers Association and the Animal Protein Producers Industry voluntary ban.[44] This poses a severe risk that animals ingesting such protein may be exposed to TSE agents. The resiliency of TSE agents is remarkable. The disease's characteristics insure that any infected animal which is rendered for animal feed will likely pass on that TSE agent to the feed. The scrapie agent cannot be destroyed by boiling, is immune to ultraviolet and ionizing radiation, and resists common forms of disinfectant. Moreover, it is very resistant to inactivation by heat, and its infectivity would not be completely destroyed by rendering. [45]

As a result, the normal rendering process cannot create animal feeds capable of protecting the livestock industry from the massive introduction of scrapie and other TSE agents into existing herds. Studies show that TSE agents may not be destroyed by maintaining continual temperatures as high as 360 Celsius.[46] The high temperatures would require the rendering industry to use cooking procedures and equipment not presently available.[47] Therefore, the continual use of potentially TSE contaminated animal protein from sheep and "downer" cows is the sole step within the rendering procedure in which the FDA and USDA can intervene in order to protect the health of current animal herd and the meat consuming public.

Consequently, the current feeding practices within the United States animal industry make the FDA's and USDA's intervention all the more imperative. As a Center for Veterinary Medicine (CMA) memo stated, "There is a growing trend in the use of meat and bone meal for calf rations...Most is used as a protein source for high production dairy cattle and for feed lot cattle."[48] The approval of bovine growth hormone (BGH) would increase the need to place dairy cows on high energy, rendered animal protein-based diets. Furthermore, researchers continue to compile growing evidence that rendered protein may be a source of fatal BSE-like agents in United States "downer" cows, and that it may even be a potential threat to humans.

As a result, the failure of the FDA and USDA to halt the widespread feeding of potentially contaminated ruminant protein to ruminants is a violation of FFDCA and the FDA's own compliance guidelines. The current FDA guideline states, "where a rendering procedure itself raises a question of disease transmission, the ingredient may be considered adulterated under...(the FFDCA)." Clearly, the use of "downer" cows and sheep is part of the rendering procedure which raises very significant questions about animal disease transmission. For this reason, the failure of the FDA and USDA to ban the feeding of ruminant animal protein to ruminants, and to develop adequate oversight of potential BSE-like contamination of animal feeds, is contrary to the agencies own guidelines and is arbitrary and capricious and not in accordance with law.

B. The FDA Should Develop An Epidemiological Investigation To Determine The Incidences of TSE's (Especially Scrapie and BSE.) Among Ruminant Animals.

To date the USDA has tested as of 1996 approximately 2500 cattle brains to determine if a BSE-like agent has been transmitted to cattle through rendered animal feeds.[49] This process, however, has a fatal flaw; the only two risk categories of cows sampled are rabies suspect cattle that are rabies negative, and cattle over two years of age that have been given protein supplements as a large part of their diet and developed neurological diseases. Hence, the current form of the government program fails to analyze the "downer" cows implicated in Wisconsin as a possible source of the TME agent. Additionally, there are no current testing procedures available to detect TSE agents in rendered animal feeds. As a result, the FDA has implemented a flawed investigation program and has no current means of determining whether rendered animal feeds meet compliance policy guidelines 7126.24 or violate the FFDCA statutory definition of adulterated.

The only reasonable and prudent action the FDA and USDA can undertake is a comprehensive, epidemiological testing of "downer" cattle to determine the incidences of TSE infection. Moreover, only through implementation of this comprehensive study can the agencies develop a means of protecting current animal herd from infection by TSE-agents. For the reasons stated here and above, a failure to do so would be arbitrary and capricious and an abandonment of agency mandates to investigate and protect the current health and welfare of animal herds and meat consumers.

C. The FDA Should Develop an Epidemiological Investigation To Determine The Incidences of CJD Among Humans

In the past the FDA has unequivocally stated that there is no evidence that scrapie of BSE is a hazard to human health.[50]

Despite taking this position, the FDA has failed to undertake a baseline study of human CJD occurrence. Such a study could aid in determining whether a Prion-agent has already infected the meat supply in the United States. Studies indicate a typical 25% error rate in the clinical diagnosis of dementia. Thus, over a quarter of the approximate 4 million Americans diagnosed with Alzheimer's Disease may be suffering from other dementia diseases including CJD: by undertaking a statistically significant study of dementia patients to determine the real incidences of CJD the FDA could monitor whether there is a correlation to the onset of the disease in conjunction with consumption of meat or milk from ruminants. Moreover, an agency position that scrapie and BSE do not represent immediate health threats without the knowledge of CJD trends in the United States can only be described as arbitrary and capricious.

Currently, the FDA does not have a CJD monitoring program to determine the current scope of the disease in the United States. As a result of the growing concerns about the BSE and CJD link, a 1989 international workshop on BSE recommended that a method for monitoring CJD incidence in the U.S. and other countries be initiated. [51]

In order to be responsive to this potential health threat the FDA should begin to implement a responsible monitoring program to ensure the health of the public.

### AGENCY ACTION REQUESTED

The FDA and USDA is currently on notice about the potential human and animal health threats posed by scrapie and BSE. At a 1989 international roundtable on BSE a physician from the National Institutes of Health wrote, "we suggest that bonemeal not be imported from the United Kingdom, and if possible, that meat byproducts not be fed to U.S. cattle at all.[52] Moreover, the roundtable's consensus recommendations included: 1) a halt in the use of rendered meat and bonemeal supplements derived from bovine and ovine carcasses as a source of protein additive for cattle and sheep; 2) initiation of epidemiological studies to determine the incidence and prevalence of "downer cattle syndrome" to determine its relationship to BSE be immediately initiated; 3) establishment of a national bovine brain bank and 4) commencement of studies on scrapie, TME and CJD isolates in bovine species including analysis of potential infection of beef and dairy products.

It was then requested in the Petition that because of the extraordinary health threat posed to both cattle and humans by the feeding of ruminant animal protein to ruminant animals that the foregoing be immediately undertaken. Subsequently the FDA published in the Federal Register on Monday August 29, 1994 Substances Prohibited from use in animal food or feed a proposed rule and a agenda letters to manufacturers of FDA-

Regulated products. The following is a synopsis of the Federal Register regarding this and shows that the FDA agreed that there was a public health risk but then because of lobbying if failed to become law. .

## DEPARTMENT OF HEALTH AND HUMAN SERVICES

### FOOD AND DRUG ADMINISTRATION
### PROPOSED RULE

SUMMARY: The food and Drug Administration (FDA) proposes to declare that specified offal from adult (more than 12 months of age) sheep and goats is not generally recognized as safe (GRAS) for use in ruminant feed and is an unproved food additive when added to ruminant feed. Accordingly, in the absence of an approved food additive regulation or investigational exemption, the use in ruminant feed of ingredients containing specified offal from adult sheep or goats will cause the feeds to be considered adulterated within the meaning of the Federal Food, Drug, and Cosmetic Act (the act). FDA is proposing this action because the specified offal may contain the agent that causes scrapie, a transmissible spongiform encephalopathy (TSE) of sheep and goats. In the United Kingdom scrapie has been epidemiologically associated with the occurrence of bovine spongiform encephalopathy (BSE), another TSE. Because FDA cannot positively rule out a direct association between scrapie, BSE and human TSE's FDA is proposing this action to protect the health of animals and humans.

### SUPPLEMENTARY INFORMATION:

1. Background: Processed tissues from sheep and goats are used as ingredients in animal feeds. These products are derived from slaughter byproducts (slaughter inedibles) and dead, dying, diseased, and disabled (4-D) animals. The slaughter inedibles include certain offal (brain, spinal cord, spleen, thymus, tonsil, lymph nodes, or intestines) that is subject of this proposed rule. Four-D animals also contain these designated materials. Such materials are designated "specified offal's" in this proposed rule. Products which are likely to contain specified

offal include, dried meat solutes, glandular meal, meat meal, meat and bone meal, animal byproduct meal, meat meal tankage, animal digest, bone ash, bone charcoal, spent bone charcoal, cooked bone meal, and bone phosphate.

A. Processing Animal Tissues for Feed Ingredients:

Generally, feed ingredients from slaughter byproducts and dead, dying, diseased, and disabled animals are processed by rendering. Rendering involves cooking the slaughter byproducts or the whole carcasses of (4-D) animals at 240 to 290 degrees F for 20 minutes to 3 hours to separate oils, fats, and protein. [53] These rendered products are used as ingredients to provide essential nutrients in animal feed. However, there are processes other than rendering, such as drying, in which slaughter byproducts are manufactured into feed ingredients.

The agent responsible for the transmission of BSE and related TSE diseases is not well characterized. It is believed to be a cattle variant of the sheep scrapie agent. [54] [55] As explained more fully below. The occurrence of BSE in cattle has not been shown to cause a TSE disease in humans.[56] On the other hand, the possibility of a causal relationship has not been disproved. BSE has not been diagnosed in cattle in the United States.[57] However, sheep scrapie is present in the United States. Accordingly, the agency believes that the potential implications for humans as well as animal health require regulatory action to minimize the possibility for the introduction of the disease into U.S. cattle. For reasons described more fully below, FDA is proposing that any feed ingredient that contains specified offal from adult sheep or goats is a food additive when added to the feed of ruminants.

B. Transmissible Spongiform Encephalopathies (TSE's)

TSE's are progressively degenerative central nervous system (CNS) diseases of man and animals that are characterized by a long incubation period, a relatively short clinical course of neurological signs, and a 100-percent mortality[58] TSE's are believed to be caused by abnormal isoform neuronal membrane proteins which contain no detectable nucleic acids, are resistant to most methods of sterilization, and survives severe environmental conditions such as 360 degrees C dry heat.[59] [60] The agent, however, is not generally believed to be a virus, but rather a protein devoid of nucleic acid components. Nucleic acid components are characteristic of other living microorganisms. These proteins have been termed prions, and are abnormal forms of proteins already present in all animals. [61] [62]

Antemortem diagnostic tests for the detection of TSE do not exist. Postmortem tests are required to confirm suspected TSE cases. The observation histopathological changes in the brain, such as vacuolization of the brainstem, are positive indicators.[63]

### 1. Sheep Scrapie

Scrapie is characterized by a prolonged incubation period averaging 2 years, followed by a clinical course of 2 to 6 months when the animal exhibits sensory and motor malfunction, depression, and death. The agent presumably moves from infected to susceptible animals by direct or indirect contact and enters through the gastrointestinal tract. Consequently, its spread is both vertical (mother to offspring in utero) and horizontal (direct contact) between sheep. Early signs of scrapie include subtle changes in behavior or temperament which may be followed by scratching and rubbing against fixed objects. Other signs include subtle changes in behavior or temperament which may be followed by scratching and rubbing against fixed objects. Other signs include loss of coordination, weight loss despite a good appetite, biting of feet and limbs, tremor around head and neck, and unusual walking habits. Since there is no detectable immune response to scrapie, diagnosis of scrapie in live sheep is possible only when clinical signs are evident and must be confirmed by histopathology at postmortem.[64]

The scrapie agent may be identified in lymphatic tissue (spleen, thymus, tonsil, and lymph nodes) in sheep, the agent is identified in the intestines, nervous tissues (brain and spinal cord), and lymphatic tissues.[65] The brain has been shown to contain by far the highest scrapie infectivity of any body tissue.

The first case of scrapie in the United States was diagnosed in Michigan in 1947. At the present time, there are 108 known scrapie-infected flocks (flocks with sheep diagnosed with scrapie) containing a total of 7,430 sheep, and there are 13 known scrapie-source flocks (flocks to which scrapie-infected sheep were traced) containing a total of 3,418 sheep. [66]

## 2. Bovine Spongiform Encephalopathy (BSE)

BSE is a transmissible, slowly progressive, degenerative disease of the CNS of adult cattle. This disease has a prolonged incubation period in cattle following oral exposure (2-8 years) and is always fatal. BSE is characterized by abnormalities of behavior, sensation, posture, and gait. The clinical signs usually begin with changes in animal behavior that are suggestive of apprehension, anxiety, and fear. There is increased reaction to sound and touch. A swaying gait is sometimes coupled with high stepping of the feet and is most evident in the hind limbs. Changes in the normal behavior of the individual cow may also include separation from the rest of the herd while at pasture, disorientation, or excessive licking of the nose or flanks. The most common history given by the herdsman was nervousness or altered behavior or temperament, weakness associated with pelvic limb ataxia, paresis, and loss of body weight.

C. Association Between Scrapie and BSE

In 1981-1982, the rendering industry in the United Kingdom reduced the use of hydrocarbon solvent extraction in the rendering process. The appearance of BSE in the United Kingdom approximately 3 years after the change in the rendering process is consistent with the 2- to 8-year incubation period of BSE. The epidemiological evidence has suggested that changes in the solvent extraction process was the major factor responsible for initiating a BSE epidemic in the United Kingdom. Furthermore, laboratory tests based on intracerebral injection studies in rodents indicated that the hydrocarbon extraction method inactivated the causative agent while the heat method did not inactivate the scrapie-like agent present in the rendered animal byproducts.[67] [68] The heat extraction method is the most common rendering process currently in use world wide.

Historical Efforts to Control BSE

United Kingdom Regulatory Actions: Regulatory controls taken to manage the BSE epidemic in the United Kingdom and to address public health concern include: (1) An action in June 1988 to make the disease reportable; (2) a ban in July 1988 on the feeding of ruminant-derived protein supplements to other ruminants; (3) an order in August 1988 for the compulsory slaughter and incineration of BSE suspect cattle; (4) a ban in November 1988 on the human consumption of specified offal's (including brain, spinal cord, thymus, spleen, tonsils, and intestines) of ruminants; and (5) a ban in September 1990 of feeding any ingredient containing specified offal's to all pet and farm animals.

United States Regulatory Actions: The USDA Animal and Plant Health Inspection Service (APHIS) has had a scrapie control program in effect since 1952. This program has been responsible for the relatively low incidence of the disease in United States. (My comment is that this has recently been repealed which does not make common sense, and I believe the entire flock should be slaughtered if a case of scrapie is found in order to wipe out this coming dreaded plague.)

To decrease further the incidence of scrapie and the threat of BSE in the United States, APHIS in 1992, initiated a voluntary certification program for sheep. Flocks that have not had a diagnosed case of scrapie within 5 years, or a case traced back to the flock in that period, may apply for APHIS certification and be officially identified as such. This new control effort provides a mechanism to recognize flocks as scrapie-free in the absence of a live animal diagnostic test.

Voluntary Ban by Renderers: In 1989, the National Renderers Association (NRA) and the Animal Protein Producers Industry (APPI) recommended to its members that they stop rendering adult sheep or sheep offal for sale as meat and bone meal for inclusion in cattle feed.[69] Following adoption of the voluntary ban, the FDA carried out a survey of current practices in the United States for rendering or otherwise disposing of adult sheep carcasses and parts, specifically head, brain, and spinal cord. Limited inspections of rendering plants were conducted to: (1)Assess compliance by United States renderers with the industry imposed voluntary ban on rendering adult sheep for cattle feed; (2) identify rendering plant practices concerning adult sheep; and (3) determine if rendered adult sheep protein byproducts were being sold or labeled for use as feed or feed components for cattle. Of the 19 plants surveyed, 15 rendered carcasses or offal of adult sheep. These 15 plants processed more than 85 percent of the adult sheep rendered in the United States. Eleven of the 15 rendered carcasses of adult sheep with heads, 7 of the 15 rendered sheep carcasses separately from other species, 6 of the 15 maintained meat and bone meal from adult sheep separate from meat and bone meal from other species, and 4 of the 15 rendered sheep that had died of causes other than slaughter. Six of the 11 renderers processing adult sheep with heads had sold meat and bone meal to manufacturers of cattle feed; thus, the rendering industry's voluntary ban was not fully implemented at the time of the survey.

Food additive Status of Specified Offal From Adult Sheep and Goats: FDA recognizes that the processed slaughter byproducts and dead, dying, diseased, and disabled animals of adult sheep and goats have a long history of use in animal feeds without known adverse effects. However, the evidence for the development of a new pattern of disease transmission now indicates that these ingredients can no longer be categorically regarded as safe. The Agency believes that the epidemiological evidence linking the occurrence of BSE in ruminants with the feed ingredients containing specified offal from adult sheep and goats precludes any claim of reliance upon a general recognition of safety as a sufficient basis for the continued use of these specified offal's in food.

The FDA reached this conclusion in light of the findings regarding a possible mechanism for the transmission of BSE to ruminants as a result of feed ingredients containing specified offal from scrapie-infected adult sheep and goats, as discussed in this document. FDA cannot determine what level of feed ingredients from processed adult sheep and goat products, if any, is safe in ruminant feed.

A search of the scientific literature did not reveal information that would provide a basis for the GENERALLY RECOGNIZED AS SAFE (GRAS) status of feed ingredients derived from processed adult sheep or goat slaughter byproducts. Nor is the agency aware of a prior sanction for any feed products that contain these products.

In view of the above, FDA has preliminary concluded that the addition of specified offal to ruminant feed constitutes, in light of the epidemiological evidence about BSE, the use of an disapproved food additive. A regulation for the use of processed adult sheep- and goat-specified offal in ruminant feed is not in effect. Therefore, it is FDA's preliminary conclusion that any ruminant feed that contain such an ingredient is adulterated. Accordingly, FDA is proposing to list specified offal from sheep or goat over 12 months of age in 21 CFR Part 589--Substances Prohibited From Use in Animal Food or Feed.

Description of the Proposed Rule: The proposed rule would prohibit use of any feed ingredient containing specified offal from sheep and goats over 12 months of age in ruminant feed. Specified offal is defined as any tissue from the brain, spinal cord, spleen, thymus, tonsil, lymph nodes, or intestines (duodenum to anus, inclusive) of sheep or goats or any processed product that is reasonably expected to contain specified offal.

## WHAT HAPPENED?

The petition was filed in 1993 by Jeremy Rifkin, in 1994 the above was published in the Federal Register that proposed a ban on using sheep offal as cattle feed, but vehement protests from the rendering and livestock industries blocked it. The Dairy and Agriculture lobbyist are among the strongest in Washington and the Golden Rule prevails. He that has gold rules. The FDA promises a ban any day now even though the proposal was published in the Federal Register, November 1994. But as you read the proposal it did not affect cattle cannibalism: some 14 percent (by weight) of the cow carcasses rendered in U.S. are fed to other cattle according to the USDA. American farmers routinely feed rendered sheep and cattle to their cows, just as the British did until scientists began suspecting that herds were getting BSE from sheep that had scrapie (Mad Sheep disease). Dr. Richard Marsh, a virologist, of the University of Wisconsin says "Eventually this practice is going to get us into trouble, we will be in the same quagmire as Great Britain." The British press is carrying prediction that 500,000 to one million beef eaters a year could die of CJD the human equivalent of the mad-cow disease.

## MAD COW DISEASE IN THE U.S.? Don't panic, but one version's already here.

That was the headlines in the medicine section of Newsweek April 8, 1996. "Most ominous, the Health Ministry announced the latest in a series of CJD deaths that are so different from the textbook description of the disease—the victims were young, the brain tissue looked like Alzheimer"s—that they suggest a link to mad cow says Dr. Paul Brown of the U.S. National Institutes of Health."

The Wall Street Journal, March 28, 1996, reported that Will Hueston, an official of the department's Animal and Plant Health Inspection Service as saying "Most of the rendering techniques they use in Britain they got from the U.S.; so there's nothing different in the range of methods." Government officials have begun to rethink the adequacy of their safeguards. The question facing the U.S. rendering industry is whether the practice of heating animal parts at 250 degrees Fahrenheit for an hour is sufficient to inactivate the likely infectious agents of BSE, called prions. Nobody knows whether the process kills prions. But as you have read previously in this chapter the proposal from the FDA they definitely stated that it wouldn't. We have to depend on our FDA and the USDA and if they cannot get congress to act then we too will not believe what the Government is telling us, just like the majority of Britain's don't believe their Government told them the truth. Officials in London have tried to quell public anxiety by denying that BSE posed a threat to public health, but the British aren't buying it. Surveys show that only 2 percent believe what their government tells them about the food they eat. And in the case of BSE, much of what the British government has asserted in the past has turned out to be wrong. In the United States the official government position is that BSE has not infected American cattle, but some scientist who have studied the disease believe otherwise.

The British government set up the Southwood Commission and they reported in 1988, "From present evidence it is likely that cattle will prove to be a 'dead-end host' for the disease agent and most unlikely that BSE will have any implications for human health. Nevertheless, if our assessments of these likelihood's are incorrect, the implications would be extremely serious." It turned out that the commission's assessments were incorrect; BSE can infect other mammals. To this day, however, British Officials continue to assert that the beef supply is fit for human consumption and can be eaten safely by everyone.

In a 1989 study at the University of Pittsburgh, three cases of CJD, that turned up in their study, had a much longer course than is usually seen with that condition and failed when the patient was alive to show the usual EEG abnormalities. In other words, the CJD cases discovered in Pittsburgh exhibited symptoms that were more compatible with Alzheimer's disease than a classic case of CJD. The Pittsburgh study could indicate that some of the 4 million people in the United States suffering from Alzheimer's may actually be infected with the agent that causes CJD. And that raises this question: has an unrecognized form of BSE infected U.S. cattle and entered the human food chain? U.S. cows that are inoculated in a laboratory with scrapie-infected sheep brain don't go mad like the British Mad Cow Disease, they simply fall down and die. This is what downer cows do. The cow falls down and either is sent to the slaughterhouse, where they are readied for human consumption, or to the rendering plant, where they end up as high-protein animal feed.

The FDA and the USDA and the committees on agriculture in the House of Representatives and the Senate are apparently ignoring any evidence that suggests that U.S. cattle are infected with BSE. They are ignoring Richard Marsh, a veterinary scientist at the University of Wisconsin. They have apparently decided that the type of BSE that appeared in Britain was the only form of the disease to be concerned about. Further, sounding very much like their British counterparts USDA officials state that the American Public has nothing to worry about, the beef in the United States, and that it is safe as no BSE has been found in American Cattle.[70]

Ironically the USDA canceled the "Scrapie Eradication Program"—which was designed to rid the U.S. of the disease—and replaced it with a scrapie-control program that was "entirely voluntary." According to the USDA , the eradication program was replaced because of cost, poor producer cooperation and failure to adequately control scrapie." Having been a Dairy and Milk Inspector for 15 years I know that human nature won't let it work. .

The USDA and the FDA, which regulate animal feed products, have decided to not interfere with beef and dairy industry practice of feeding dead cows to living cows. The APHIS explains, is "that the cost to the livestock and rendering industries would be substantial" and that such a change in policy "could pose major problems for the U.S. livestock and rendering industries." Consequently greed from corporate interests has won out over the interest of public health.

### A NEW PLAGUE?

Now some evidence indicates that spongiform encephalopathy has appeared in the U.S. cattle population.

In response to mounting public fears, Britain's Ministry of Agriculture, Fisheries and Forestry reported in 1989 that BSE posed no public health threat because cows were a "dead-end host" and could not transmit the disease to other animals. But this was not the case. BSE has been shown to be easily transmitted to other mammals by laboratory experiments. In fact mice, pigs, sheep, goats and monkeys whose brains were inoculated with Mad Cow infected material developed spongiform encephalopathies. In Great Britain, pet cats, some zoo animals, including the eland, oryx, cheetahs and pumas developed their type of Mad Cow disease from eating contaminated food from Mad Cows.

Now evidence suggest that the Mad Cow disease has already been transmitted to humans and that this new variant of the Mad Cow Disease even affects the very young, teens as well as older people. In March 1993 a dairy farmer had died of

CJD who had drunk milk from his dairy herd for the seven years prior to 1989. That was the year some cows in his herd developed mad cow disease and were incinerated.

Michael Hansen, a biologist employed as a research associate at Consumers Union testified at a public hearing, by the FDA's Veterinary Medicine Advisory Committee, to take testimony about bovine growth hormone, that when injected into cows, increases their milk production. Hansen was concerned that when milk production is artificially increased, cows will require more protein supplements made from the rendered carcasses of cows and sheep. Hansen challenged the federal government's official line that no cases of BSE have been documented in the United States. He then advised the committee that some American cattle may already be infected with BSE. He referred to the mink ranch in Stentsonville, Wis., that was wiped out by the transmissible mink encephalopathy (Mad Mink disease) because their diet consisted of 95% downer cows." Dr. Richard Marsh believes that some downer cows are afflicted with a milder type of the Mad Cow disease in the United States and has already infected the U.S. cattle population. He said that Mad Cow disease cattle, in Europe, went mad prior to dying, but BSE-infected cows in the U.S. simply fell down and died. Each year in the U.S. about 100,000 cattle die from the downer cow syndrome. Marsh believes the widespread practice of feeding cows to living cows should be outlawed. He is trying to inform farmers not to use ruminants (cows and cud chewing animals) to be used for animal protein feed. Many dairymen do not even know they are feeding dead cows to their cows. Marsh and Hansen are concerned about the lukewarm federal response which is a serious public health threat. The USDA has done nothing to stop this practice. The USDA tends to respond to commodity groups rather than consumers, and the government hasn't taken any measures to restrict what goes into animal feed.[71]

Mr. Douglas Hogg, the agriculture minister of Great Britain believes that since there has still been cases of BSE in cows born after the ruminant feed ban of July 1988, that there has been some continued leakage of BSE infected material into animal

feed. As of July 19, 1995 20,219 cases of BSE has been confirmed in cattle born after the feed ban and he contributes these
cases to a food-borne source of infection.[72]

Patterson reports in the Journal of Public Health Medicine
in 1995 that even though the feeding of animal protein of ruminant origin to ruminants was prohibited in July 1988 it is now
know that this ruminant feed ban was not effective immediately
and that cattle born after this date continued to develop BSE. In
November 1989, almost 18 months after concern was expressed
about the possible inclusion of bovine brain, in cooked products,
such as meat pies, specified bovine offal's (brain, spinal cord,
gut, tonsil, thymus and spleen) were eventually excluded from
the human diet. But before this measure, many in Britain were
exposed to potentially infected Mad Cow meat. Cattle up to six
months of age were exempt from the ban which was a grave
mistake, because it has now been demonstrated that BSE is
transmissible to laboratory mice from the intestines of young
cattle, slaughtered just six-months after oral challenge with the
BSE agent.[73] A complete ban on the sale of all bovine offal
products prepared from animals under six months old had earlier
been recommended in May 1990. However, it was July 1994
before the ban was partially extended to include the intestines
and thymus of cattle under six months of age, but not the remaining specified bovine offal's. We see that the goal-posts in
the control of Mad Cow disease are changing. Should they
move again, public confidence in food safety may be irreparably
damaged.[74]

In Britain, beef cattle are normally slaughtered for human
consumption around two years of age. It is scary that the majority of infected cattle with the mad cow disease will have been
slaughtered before the onset of clinical disease. Clinical disease
lasts two weeks to six months and is diagnosed by observing
nervousness, kicking, abnormal gait and leg instability. If not
destroyed, affected animals develop a swaying gait, weight loss
and behavioral problems. Injuries are common because of re-
peated falling. Death is preceded by an inability to stand and
coma.[75]

In CJD the human TSE type of Mad Cow disease is characterized by a rapidly progressive dementia, movement disorder and death. Usually it is most common between 55 and 75 years of age. The median duration of illness is only four months and 90 per cent of patients survive less than one year.

## SUMMARY

The dilemma remains today even in the United States that much of the debate regarding controls to protect the public health has become polarized and politicized. This has been un-helpful. It is imperative that public health doctors are encouraged to contribute to what many regard as the most serious public health problem to face us in recent years. BSE must not become an area in which angels fear to tread. As it has been in the past, the Medical doctors tended to humans and knew very little about veterinary medicine. The USDA even though composed mainly of Veterinary doctors, in most scenarios, were using their energies to protect the Agriculture industry, and when ever it was asked about the dangers of a possible health problem, regarding animal diseases to humans, the answer was that the disease could not jump species and that it is not SCIENTIFICALLY sound or not proven. Even today with our Epidemiology it is not possible to prove the etiology of many human diseases because of our lack of sensitive specialized tests. This is changing with the PCR (polymerase chain reaction test) test and mapping of the human genome.

In the United States where we are making the same mistake as the British did in feeding cattle and sheep that have the Mad Sheep disease to cattle as protein rations to increase milk production and fatten beef cattle. There can be no dispute that the human food chain in Britain has become contaminated with the BSE agent. In the U.S. it may have, and once we know for sure, it will be too late to do anything about it, to prevent humans from getting a form of the Mad Cow disease.(Cruetzfeldt-Jakob disease).

In Britain most of the apparently healthy cattle that are infected with the Mad Cow disease will have entered the human food chain. In Britain by the time the first obviously sick cows

63

were detected, many thousands of cattle were already incubating the disease. The inability to neutralize the Mad Cow agent effectively during food processing and cooking means that, in all probability, most humans who have consumed beef since the start of the Mad Cow epidemic will have been exposed to the agent. The same thing may be happening in the U.S. Since the BSE agent is new, has not been isolated or identified, causes fatal disease by an unknown mechanism, can infect a range of animal species and is highly resistant to sterilization. Because of this we must stop feeding sheep and cows to cows like we are doing in the United States today. It only makes common sense. It will be many years before we can be confident that the public health has not been compromised and that diseases that the etiology is unknown like Alheizemers may be related to feeding Ruminants to Ruminants. Other stupid practices involved in feeding cows was brought out in Hoards Dairyman June 1993, the National Dairy Magazine by Greg Fetter who said "And cows will eat darn near everything" That includes banana skins, dried and ground. "There is also dried poultry waste. Yes, processed chicken poop sells for $45 a ton. And the cows eat it. Or the dairyman can order "feather meal"... which is just what it sounds like—meal made of ground chicken or turkey feathers." When I took Feeds and Feeding at California State Polytechnic College at San Luis Obispo, California, we were taught to feed the cows a ration that didn't include meat. Today they may be fed bakery products, such as day-old donuts, bread and cookies. Sometimes their feed includes garbage from restaurants.

The FDA should rule in the interest of the safety of the consumer rather than the safety of the beef industry. The World Health Organization recommended a ban on ruminant feed at the conclusion of their meeting in April of 96. WHO has thoroughly studied the problem yet America continues to back pedal, requiring more petitions and repetitious research.

# CHAPTER THREE

# RECENT NEWS FLASHES

In researching this material about the mad cow disease I became convinced that it was imperative that the information be taken seriously. I decided to take a leave of absence from my medical practice and work full time on getting the facts about this disease available to the public. The potential health risk to all consumers of milk, meat, gelatin, or other products derived from cattle needed to be explored. While working on this information, the whole situation of the mad cow disease exploded in Britain, with shock waves reverberating to include Europe, Australia, India, Argentina, and United States. Daily the television showed pictures of staggering cattle, angry consumers, and solemn scientists. The whole situation was explored in the media. I have recorded chronologically the information as it was given on Reuters news agency. This is a mirror of what can happen in the United States if we ignore the potential for disaster in our current feeding practices.

### WORLD SHOCKED BY MAD COWS

12/6/95 - LONDON   Hundreds of British schools on Wednesday pulled beef off dinner menus under pressure from parents who fear "mad cow" disease can give humans a deadly illness. The government insisted that the scare about infected beef was exaggerated and ministers urged people to keep eating beef, but nine out of 10 people in a television phone  poll said they did not believe the government.   Beef sales have fallen by five percent. Several dairy farmers and two adolescents have died from Creutzfeldt-Jakob disease (CJD), a degenerative infection that turns the brain spongy, and kills all its victims. Agriculture Minister David Hogg visited London's historic Smithfield Market to insist that beef was not dangerous. Posing for cameras among lines of carcasses, he said. "I am absolutely certain that British beef is wholly safe."

12/6/95 LONDON Two local government bodies banned beef from their menus, because of growing worries that people can catch a deadly brain disease from infected beef. Fears about BSE or mad cow disease have risen across Britain after reports of several deaths of adolescents and dairy workers from the human version of the killer illness. Schools said they were besieged by demands from parents to stop serving beef to their children. "we are mindful of parents' concerns and have acted accordingly," said Bet Jenkins, head of catering for schools in West's Glamorgan, Wales. "The majority of our primary schools have now taken beef from their menus." Colin Blakemore, professor of physiology at Oxford University told the Times newspaper: "I stopped eating beef as soon as the first BSE scare was made public in 1986." Tim Lang, Professor of Food Policy at Thames Valley University and former director of the Parents for Safe Food Campaign, said he had stopped eating beef products six years ago and would not allow small children to do so. Brain surgeon Sir Bernard Tomlinson said he would not eat products such as beefburgers "under any circumstances, nor would I eat beef liver or meat pies."

3/6/96 BONN - German scientist said Britain must have failed to carry out proper measures to stop "mad cow disease spreading in herds, unless the disorder was raging in a way experts have not yet established. Britain banned the use of cattle innards that scientists think can harbor Bovine Spongiform Encephalopathy from all animal feeds in 1990, two years after banning the use of cattle remains in cattle feed.

3/20/96 LONDON - The British government said today

for the first time that the so-called mad cow disease, a lethal brain condition, could probably be transmitted to humans. Health Secretary Stephen Dorrell said an advisory committee of scientists and doctors had concluded that 10 people who died from Creutzfeldt-Jakob Disease (CHD) probably caught it from beef that was infected before the government introduced safety measures on the handling of meat in 1989. Until today the government had refused to accept the possibility that BSE can jump species and trigger CJD which is extremely rare in humans but always fatal.

3/21/96 LONDON - Fears that humans can catch "mad cow" disease stampeded Britain's European partners into banning British beef. Alarm bells rang when Britain said it had found a likely link between "mad cow" disease and its human equivalent. Scientists are meeting in Britain this weekend to decide whether children were more at risk than adults. Hundreds of schools in Britain have already taken beef off their menus. Dorrell's statement reversed 10 years of government assurances that BSE was not linked to its human equivalent. The new findings by government-appointed scientists followed studies of 10 young people who died from the degenerative brain disease which can take more than 10 years to show itself. Officials say those who died of CJD had probably contracted the disease before the safety measures intended to prevent BSE from entering the human food chain were introduced in 1989. The government U-turn prompted many Britons to ask whether ministers could be trusted. Consumer groups attacked British policy. The Brussels-based European consumer association, said the British government should have acted much earlier. "The delay is inexcusable," Director Jim Murray said.

3/21/96 WASHINGTON DC - Will Hueston, a spokesman for the United States Department of Agriculture, said that U.S. officials have tested the brains of 2,791 cattle in the United States, including some British cattle imported before the ban, and have found no evidence of the disease.

3/21/96 PARIS - France rejected a British complaint that a ban on British beef imports was illegal and vowed to keep the suspension going until fears over mad cow disease had been lifted. French farm minister Philippe Vasseur said he was merely following scientific advice. "If the scientist tell me there is still some doubt, we will keep our health cordon in place. If the scientists tell me the doubt has been lifted, then trade can resume.

3/21/96 LONDON - Doug Eland, a partner at Peter Tocher butchers, said the new scare could not have come at a worst time. This has happened in the run-up to Easter. Eland blamed the government for botching the announcement. "Just look at this," he said, brandishing a copy of the left-leaning Daily Mirror newspaper which supported a large front-page picture of a sickly woman who died of CJD just after giving birth to a son. "They do this kind of thing because they hate the government, and I'm beginning to do so too." But butchers and farmers said it was too early yet to predict whether the crisis would be long-lasting. "The government has cried wolf for so long that people will either ignore this or it will be the straw that breaks the camel's back," said Eland.

3/21/96 LONDON - Dorrell fanned the flames of public disquiet by saying it was possible Britain's entire beef herd might be slaughtered to stop the disease in its tracks, although Agriculture Minister Douglas Hogg later seemed to play down the possibility.

3/22/96 LONDON - Steak and rib joints in central London were deserts of empty booths and tables, as panicky customers, fearful of "mad cow" disease, turned away from beef to eating chicken and fish instead. At a popular hamburger restaurant near Leicester Square, morning staff said they had not noticed a significant drop-off in customers. By lunch time the restaurant was as usual full to bursting. But chicken pieces and vegetarian burgers were the most popular choice, according to cashiers. But some were determined not to change their eating habits. "Live it up," one building worker observed sarcastically to his friend as they waited for their orders of beefburgers. "Might as well be mad cow's disease as anything else," the friend responded, laughing.

3/22/96  LONDON  - "Could it be worse than AIDS?" The stark headline in the Daily Mail newspaper encapsulated the fear and uncertainty gripping Britain since scientists disclosed a probable link between "mad cow" disease and its human equivalent, Creutzfeldt-Jakob Disease (CJD). CJD affects humans in the same way that Bovine Spongiform Encephalopathy (BSE) makes cows mad, by eating away nerve cells in the brain until it looks like a spongy Swiss cheese. The disease is incurable. Victims show signs of dementia and memory loss and usually die within six months. Television pictures of cows frothing at the mouth and struggling to stand on wobbly legs have become sadly familiar. Doctors are at a loss to know whether this week's cases are the stirrings of a major public health catastrophe. Professor Richard Lacey, a microbiologist said "This is why we are now estimating that next century the typical number of CJD human cases will run at between 5,000 and 500,000 a year." Professor John Pattison, the chairman of a panel of scientist and doctors advising the government, speaking on Channel Four television  said,  "It could be as high as tens of thousands and, cumulatively of course, hundreds of thousands."

3/22/96  BONN - German ministers criticized their British counterparts for failing to give their European Union partners advance warning of new scientific evidence, disclosed to Parliament that humans eating mad cow-infected beef risked fatal Creutzfelt-Jakob disease and they also criticized British measures to protect consumers as inadequate. Agriculture Minister Jochen Borchert presented a list of draconian measures that they want the European Union to toughen existing controls. Germany wants total bans on the direct or indirect imports of British beef products and on their use in medicine and cosmetics within the European Union. Asked whether Britain should slaughter its entire herd of 11 million cattle, Seehofer said such thoughts were in his mind, but he declined to tell the British government what it should do. He was scathing about British responses, when Germany asked about the two or three cases of BSE identified in 1992 and 1993. "They said Germany was being hysterical and talked about 'German Angst' and said they must be due to old stocks of animal feed that escaped controls imposed in 1989 to prevent BSE-infected sheep brains entering the food chain.

3/22/96 - Germany, Singapore, New Zealand and Finland , France, Belgium, the Netherlands, Sweden and Portugal all halted imports of beef from Britain. Britain's own main consumer group told people to stop eating beef. Britons government admitted that it was considering mass slaughtering of cattle to eradicate mad cow disease to restore public confidence. Some British scientists have warned that up to one million people could be infected with CJD, which destroys nerve cells in the brain causing dementia, incapacity and then death.

3/22/96 AMSTERDAM - The Dutch unit of U.S. hamburger giant McDonalds Corp. said it had withdrawn 60 tons of British beef in the face of mounting customer concern over the danger of "mad cow" disease.

3/22/96 LONDON - Britain's "mad cow" disease scare sent shockwaves throughout Europe as newspapers carried headline about "Killer Steaks" and speculated how many thousands of beef consumers might eventually die. The left-of-center French daily Liberation ran the headline "Mort Aux Vaches," which literally means "Death to the Cows" but is also an old French leftist slogan meaning "Kill the Cops." It accused French officials of covering up what it alleged was a long-standing practice of importing suspect British cattle to Brittany to be resold labeled as French. In Italy the scare made the front page of all major newspapers. "mad cow Disease, Terror in Europe," Corriere della Sera said in a headline. "European alarm over killer meat," said the Turin newspaper La Stampa.

The Bonn-based daily General Anzeiger said the British government has had to admit that it lost sight of the well-being of its own people and other Europeans for the sake of short-term economic benefits. A commentator on German ARD television said there could only be one decision: "Not one gram of beef should be allowed to be exported anymore. Now the health of the consumer must take absolute precedence. The interests of British meat producers should no longer play a role." In Belgium, Lq Derniere Heure newspaper said in a headline, "Stop the Meat that Kills" next to a large photograph of a cow with a black strip across its eyes—a technique normally reserved for criminal mug shots. In Austria, the mass-circulation Kurier newspaper fronted the story with a report saying Scottish experts feared between 5,000 and 15,000 people could be infected.

3/22/96 GENEVA - Dr. Lindsay Martinez from the World Health Organization said that many unanswered questions remained about the new form of CJD. It has struck younger patients, lasts twice as long, seems to have no hereditary link, and affects the brain differently from the classical CJD. "We may still see more cases in the future, because I don't know how long the incubation period might be, so there may still be other individuals who are unfortunately in the incubation period and will go on to develop the disease. But that is from an earlier exposure, not from a recent one.

3/22/96 MOSCOW - Russia's chief veterinary inspector said that they stopped importing British beef six years ago because we knew they have Bovine leucosis (leukemia) and BSE in British beef.

3/22/96 AMMAN—Jordan suspended imports of British dairy products and Irish livestock. Health Minister Batayneh said Jordan had not imported any dairy products or livestock from Ireland since 1990.

3/22/96 HELSINKI Finland on Friday joined countries banning imports of British beef in response to scientists discovery of a likely link between mad cow disease and its fatal human equivalent.

3/22/96    SINGAPORE—Singapore and New Zealand joined a handful of European countries in banning British beef on Friday after the UK's livestock industry was devastated by a report that mad cow disease may be able to jump to humans. New Zealand suspended imports containing material from British cattle, including cooked and canned meat, gelatin which may be made out of cattle hides, meat pastes, lard, sausage rolls, and meat imported for use on airline flights. Graham Roberson, president of the Federated Farmers lobby Group, said many farmers believed the government should not even run the risk of importing bovine genetic material.

3/22/96  BONN—Germany said today it was banning all imports of British beef in connection with fears that it could infect humans with so-called mad cow disease. There were four cases of BSE in Germany last year, and the farmers' association says they all involved cattle imported from Britain.

3/23/96  SEOUL - South Korea banned imports on Saturday of any beef and cattle bone powder from Britain. So far this year, South Korea has imported about 37,400 tons of beef from the United States, Australia, New Zealand and Canada, and about 180 tons of cattle bone powder from Russia, France and Bangladesh, government figures showed.

3/23/96  BRUSSELS - Switzerland recorded around 160 cases of mad cow disease between 1986-96 said Jean Girardin, Farmers Union representative in Brussels. Switzerland is after Britain the European country most affected by BSE.

3/23/96  BONN - Germany has imposed a ban on beef from Switzerland because this is the main country apart from Britain where cases of BSE have occurred in home-reared cattle. Bonn as already asked its regional states to order farmers to slaughter all 5,000 or so cattle imported from Britain.

3/23/96  PARIS  - French rightist politician Philippe de Villiers is suing the European Commission, charging that it concealed evidence for years that mad cow disease could affect humans.  "I am saying that the Brussels Commission was aware that there were indications that the mad cow disease could be transmitted to man," he told the weekly Journal du Dimanche in an interview to be published tomorrow.  "We accuse the Commission of covering up or ignoring information it has had for 10 years, because we also accuse it of hampering the state protection of consumers for the sake of the free movement of goods."

3/24/96  LISBON - The current mad cow scare underlines a lack of sanitary controls in Portugal where meat was consumed that may have been contaminated with the agent that causes the disease, a Lisbon daily reported.  The newspaper had said that meat-based feed used for cattle in Portugal could have been exposed to the agent which causes the disease because of inadequate checks on its origin. Lisbon has also ordered closer monitoring of cattle in Portugal where  27 cases of the disease have been reported  The infected animals were slaughtered along with any with which they had been in contact.

3/24/96 DUBLIN - Ireland, a major beef producer, said it would back a European Union ban on British beef exports because of its "mad cow" disease scare. A growing number of countries outside the 15 - nation bloc have also banned British beef, including New Zealand, South Africa, Singapore, Cyprus and Egypt.  Some Irish farmers had sold blank health certificates to British farmers to help them get round the scare caused by BSE. "That story is broadly correct" said Agriculture Minister Ivan Yates. "But false certification has stopped. It's appalling and unacceptable activity and we have no evidence that it is widespread."  Yates said there had been 124 cases of BSE in Irish herds over the past six and a half years compared to 160,000 in Britain.  But he said Irish policy was to slaughter entire herds where one animal was found infected

· with BSE whereas in Britain only the sick animal was killed.

3/25/96 SAN JOSE, Costa Rica - Costa Rican customs officials yesterday searched bags belonging to European tourists for beef in an effort to quell fears over the introduction of mad cow disease.

3/25/96 LONDON - Newspapers reserved their ire for British Prime Minister John Major's decision not to order mass slaughter of cattle to restore confidence in the four billion pound (6 billion) beef industry. "The government comes out of this badly... they were guilty—as so often before—of pathetic public relations," stormed the Sun newspaper. "Unless John Major is very careful, casualty figures for slaughtered Tories on election day will exceed deaths caused by eating beef from mad cows," it wrote. Major has a majority of just two in parliament and must call an election by next May. During an ill - tempered debate on the government's decision not to slaughter large numbers of cattle which might have BSE , or "mad cow" disease, one Conservative parliamentarian called Labor health spokeswoman Harrier Harman a "stupid cow." He was immediately forced to withdraw his remark.

3/25/96 COPENHAGEN - Denmark said it planned to ban British beef imports if the European Union did not agree on a general ban because of the mad cow disease.

3/25/95 CAIRO - Egyptian President Hosni Mubarak, who last week banned imports of European meat, revealed in an interview that he did not eat red meat and advised other Egyptians to follow his example. "There are alternative solutions. I would like to mention here that meat is not everything as far as the dinner table is concerned. Too much of it is harmful to the health. I, for example don't eat red meat at all in any form." Two ships carrying 3,600 Irish cattle have left Egyptian territorial waters on orders from the Egyptian authorities.

3/25/96 WASHINGTON DC - Agriculture Secretary Dan

Glickman that the United States would give technical assistance to Britain to try to combat so-called mad cow disease. Glickman said that the nature of the disease and its popular name had contributed to "excessive sensationalism and we'll probably end up finding that it's not quite as widespread as the British press is talking about."

3/25/96 BRUSSELS - Belgian farmers will patrol the country's ports to prevent British beef from being imported, a farmers' union spokesman said. "There is a ban but the past has taught us that quite often things of which imports were banned still got in," the spokesman of the General Farmers' Syndicate said.

3/25/96 BRUSSELS - European Union Agriculture Commissioner Franz Fischler confirmed a vote by European Union officials to ban exports of British beef and cattle products because of concern over mad cow disease. Fischler said the ban extends to live animal sperm, and embryos, and meat of cattle which have been slaughtered or will be slaughtered in Britain. It also covers meat products used for medicinal, pharmaceutical, and cosmetic purposes. "Exports from the UK of meat and other related products are now banned," Fischler said.

3/25/96 LONDON - Britain's cattle farmers braced for a shattering blow to their industry on Monday as experts pondered drastic measures to deal with mad cow disease. The government, widely criticized for doing too little too late to tackle a crisis that has sparked worldwide alarm, could announce the slaughter of one third of Britain's 11 -million cattle herd to try to root out the disease. There is concern that children, who eat millions of beefburgers every year, could be particularly at risk. The government had refused to countenance such a link for 10 years despite growing public concern.

3/25/96 CHICAGO - Wendy's International Inc. Will stop serving British beef in its eight restaurants in the United Kingdom due to possible concerns regarding "mad cow" disease in that country, the company said today. Wendy's has a total of 4,800 restaurants worldwide. McDonald's Corp. Also has taken beef off its menu at its 660 restaurants in Britain and will resume serving beef in three days from Dutch supplies.

3/25/96 PARIS - A herd of 151 cattle was slaughtered on Monday after a rare case of mad cow disease in France, which led European nations in banning imports of British beef last week to stem the spread of contamination. A second herd of 120 cattle will be slaughtered on April 1 in northwestern France, said Loic Gouello, head of veterinary services in the Cotes d'Armor region of Brittany. Every time a case has been found in France, the entire herd has been slaughtered and incinerated. A single animal was detected in each case Gouello said. The next herd to be slaughtered had apparently consumed bone meal made from ground up parts of infected animals before a ban was imposed in 1989, he said.

3/25/96 WASHINGTON DC - At a meeting of the U.S. Agriculture Department, Gary Weber, from the National Cattlemen's Beef Association said there just isn't enough information to say whether the brain disease CJD should be linked to mad cow. There are only 109 head of cattle from Britain in the United States. These animals are monitored every six months for any signs of BSE. They are used only for breeding purposes and will never enter the food chain.

3/25/96 BANGKOK - Thailand is to destroy all unauthorized imports of beef products for fear of the mad cow disease, a government official said today.

3/25/96 LONDON - Agriculture secretary Douglas Hogg said bans of British beef imports initiated by many countries last week were unjustified, and he made no mention of the slaughter of the national cattle herd, a step he said previously was under consideration.

3/26/95 TOKYO - The Japanese government extended a ban on British beef to include food products such as sausages and canned meat because of fears over mad cow disease.

3/26/96 LONDON - Britain appeared to be fighting a losing battle to persuade the European Union to lift an export ban on its beef and convince consumers worldwide they were not at risk from the human form of "mad cow" disease. "Believe the evidence. Don't get swept up in the hysteria," British Health Minister Stephen Dorrell urged consumers. The scare he sparked had spread worldwide. Irish police were patrolling the border with Northern Ireland, to stop unscrupulous farmers trying to smuggle their cattle classed as British—into Ireland for export. Britain's top consumer body attacked Dorrell for calling consumers "mad" for refusing to eat British beef. "The Government has failed to provide scientific proof one way or the other and it is reasonable to expect people to want to protect themselves and their children," said Consumer's Association spokesman Steve Harris.

3/26/96 BRUSSELS - Farmers visited deep-freeze warehouses, slaughterhouses and the premises of meat importers at Belgium's leading ports and reported suspicious consignments of beef from Britain to the authorities. As well as a ban by countries, British farmers also face a growing boycott by food providers ranging from fast food restaurants to airlines.

3/26/96 LONDON - Prime Minister John Major said he would consider whether some of Britain's 11 million cattle should be slaughtered to allay public fears—just a day after his ministers ruled out the idea. The National Farmers Union sent a letter to the government calling on it to restore public confidence in beef by setting up a special scheme to ensure older cows did not enter the human food chain. It is vital to restore confidence in consumers not just in the United Kingdom but also throughout Europe and the rest of the world, said National Farmers' Union president Sir David Naish

3/26/96 GENEVA - The World Health Organization announce that it would host a two-day meeting of experts to study the suspected link between mad cow disease and a degenerative brain disease killing humans. The closed door talks will be held in Geneva on April 2-3. It could take up to two years of research to establish firm proof of a direct link between the new form of CJD and BSE. Unlike the classical CJD, the new form is not hereditary, has an incubation period of about 10 years, takes twice as long to kill its victims or roughly one year, and affects the brain differently, according to WHO experts.

"It is abundantly clear that measures taken so far failed to lead to the cessation of the BSE epidemic," said Arpad Somogi of the Berlin-based German Institute for the Consumer Health Protection. There are over 24,000 cases in animals that were born after the feed ban. It could be that these measures were blatantly disregarded, or there could be another source of disease." A Munich clinic said it was treating a patient suspected to have a new strain of Creutzfeldt-Jakob Disease which the British government said last week may be linked to mad cow disease. If confirmed, the case would be the first of the new strain reported in Germany. The woman worked for years in a restaurant kitchen, coming into contact with beef regularly. "These are invariably deadly diseases. One cannot sit back and contemplate academically what other proofs are needed to take more stringent measures." Somogi said.

Brain and spinal cord tissue are believed to be the chief vehicles of BSE transmission, but the scientists said they were still investigating whether it could be transmitted through the muscle tissue consumed as ordinary meat. They said it was unlikely BSE could be passed on through milk products or cosmetics manufactured with offal products. The federal government has asked the regional states to order farmers to slaughter all 5,000 or so cattle imported from Britain.

3/26/96 BRUSSELS - The European Commission cannot confirm that British beef is either safe or unsafe Lars Hoelgaard said scientific investigations to date had detected BSE or mad cow disease only in cows brains and spinal cords, but added it was possible that the only effective method for detecting BSE might be "not sensitive enough" to show low levels of infection. British liberal Graham Watson said "The public need to know the food they eat is safe. The British government is unable categorically to give that assurance.

3/26/96 LONDON - It was Hogg, with Health Secretary Stephen Dorrell, who started the crisis last week when they said scientists had found a likely link between mad cow disease and its human equivalent. The news, based on 10 cases of people suffering a new variant of the human illness, Creutzfeldt-Jakob Disease, reversed a decade of official denials of any such link. European Union Agriculture Commissioner Franz Fischler wrote to British farm minister Douglas Hogg criticizing his handling of the affair. Fischler said he was surprised Britain's representative at farm ministers' meeting on March 19 had not warned him. And in a criticism that particularly infuriated the government, Fischler said Britain's reaction had been either wrong or hasty. "If the new findings of your scientists are as troubling as they sound, then the measures you announced seem insufficient..." he wrote. "If, on the other hand... your findings do not add much to the existing body of knowledge about a link with BSE, then a more careful reaction might have been preferable.

3/26/96 VIENNA - Following the discovery of 206 cases of mad cow disease in Swiss cows, Austria banned Swiss beef and beef products, health official, Ernst Bobek said, "I presume this is because several years ago the Swiss were allowed to feed cows with animal proteins that were not sufficiently sterilized, according to my sources these were imported from the United Kingdom."

3/26/96 CHICAGO - U.S. health authorities said they are monitoring Britain's mad cow disease situation but see no reason for Americans to worry. A spokesman for CDC Bob Howard said "We have never found BSE in the United States and we have looked for it. Now, not every cow that dies in the

United States is autopsied, so you can't clearly and categorically say, 'No, it does not exist here' ... but we have never found it."

3/26/95 PARIS - French Agriculture Minister Phillips Vaster urged consumers to eat French meat and said the label guaranteed beef was safe from BSE and that cattle had been raised with vegetable feed only. The label features the letters VF for "viande francaise" (French meat) in the blue, white and red colors of the tricolor flag.

3/27/95 TAIPEI - Taiwan's Council of Agriculture will discuss a likely ban on selling dairy and canned beef products imported from Britain. We are looking into milk powder imported from Britain, which some people are concerned about due to mad cow disease.

3/27/96 LONDON - Victims of the human equivalent of "mad cow" disease face a horrific death—they go slowly mad and then die, their brains riddled with holes. Now the scientists who consistently warned diseases could jump from species to species say they are right. People who did nothing more unusual than eat a beefburger could now die, according to the latest evidence, in the same way as dwarfs who received diseased growth hormones and cannibals who ate human brains in the jungles of Papua, New Guinea. Consumers around the world have shunned British beef since scientists concluded that 10 people who died from CJD had probably caught it from beef. The cattle had in turn got the disease from sick sheep ground into fodder. Leading food researcher Peter Cox said: "In farming we have turned vegetarian cows into carnivores and then cannibals. "It's grossly unnatural and has created a timebomb which is now beginning to go off. Playing games with nature has bred a number of crises which are stacked up like planes waiting to land." There have been 70 cases of "mad cat disease" among Britain's seven million domestic cats. It has also spread to mice and pigs and zoo animals like elk, marmosets, antelopes, kudu, oryx, eland, cheetah, puma, ocelot and ostrich. CJD, like AIDS, has a long incubation period and there is no known cure. Its victims, who may have been infected up to 30 years before, die within six months of the first symptoms. They end up as virtual vegetables. It affects humans in the same way that Bovine Spongiform Encephalopathy makes cows mad by eating away nerve cells in the brain until it looks like a spongy Swiss Cheese. The CJD timebomb ticks slowly. Victims first suffer poor concentration, depression and anxiety attacks. Trembling, writhing and jerking follow. Patients become mute and incontinent. They can no longer eat.

3/27/95 LONDON - What has really shaken scientists is the possibility that eating infected meat might infect humans, a theory considered impossible until recently, and which is still treated with caution by many scientists. Some scientists have shocked the public with ominous projections. Dr. Stephen Dealler of the BSE research campaign said up to one million Britons might develop CJD, the human equivalent of mad cow disease.

3/27/95 THE HAGUE - The Netherlands said it had ordered the destruction of 64,000 British calves and was advising its consumers not to eat British beef.

3/27/96 CHICAGO - The mad cow scare, which has shut off British beef exports to Europe, may present opportunities for U.S. meatpackers, who say they can produce the non-hormone beef Europeans want. Since 1989, the European Community has banned the import of beef produced with artificial growth hormones. Much of U.S. beef is produced using such hormones, although a small number of cattle producers avoid the drugs, and their beef has been cleared for shipment to Europe. The industry estimates weight gain for hormone-treated cattle is about 10 percent faster on the same amount of feed than for untreated cattle.

3/27/96 BRUSSELS - The European Commission put the entire British beef industry in quarantine today with a temporary global export ban on all its products due to a possible threat to human health. Farm Commissioner Franz Fischler told the European Parliament, "The fact that there is no proof that there is no link is leading us to act." He said. Victims of CJD face a horrific death—they go slowly mad and then die as their brains become riddled with holes.

3/27/95 ATHENS - Greek consumers gripped by fear of mad cow disease despite a ban on British beef imports, are shunning beef in general. "Thatcher Made The Cows Mad," said the banner front-page headline in the leading Athens liberal daily Eleftherotypia. The paper claimed that the former conservative prime minister Margaret Thatcher had so relaxed British agricultural controls that plant-eating animals were fed meat, prompting the spread of the disease.

3/27/96 LONDON - Prime Minister John Major, with little choice but to embark upon an embarrassing policy U-turn, held a late-night meeting with ministers to discuss ways of tackling the crisis. Blair, leader of the main opposition Labor party, homed in for the kill in parliament. "I have to say that this matter has been handled with quite mind-boggling incompetence," he said to loud Labor cheers. Major sought to turn the blame back onto opposition parties, accusing them of helping to whip up what he said was the hysteria around mad cow disease. He said "Too often Mr. Major has held to a position long after it should have been abandoned, and then when the maximum disadvantage had accrued, he has folded."

3/28/95 JOHANNESBURG - Africans should eat their healthy bred rhinos, elephants and other wild beasts rather than follow intensive farming methods that led to mad cow disease a South African restaurateur said "One reason is these awful modern methods—pumping in steroids and hormones, dipping and now cloning. It's interfering in nature and we're bound to stuff it up sooner or later and end up with more things like mad cow disease"

3/28/96 BRUSSELS - The European Parliament said that all European Union member states, not just Britain, should introduce measures to eradicate mad cow disease. The EU ban on British beef should remain in force until this eradication plan has proved effective, it stressed, adding that the British government's failure to cull entire herds found to contain animals with BSE has played a major part in this agricultural catastrophe.

3/28/96 WASHINGTON - A Washington-based consumer group said it would sue to try and ban the feeding of rendered animal parts to cattle. "Feeding rendered sheep and cow parts to cows is an unnatural and dangerous practice," said Jeremy Rifkin, president of the Foundation on Economic Trends. The group which funds the Pure Food Campaign, said its suit would seek to compel the Food and Drug Administration to implement a ban immediately. Another consumer-oriented organization, the International Center for Technology Assessment, said it filed similar legal action against the FDA . FDA officials were not immediately available to comment on the suits.

3/28/96 LONDON - British beef is being treated like a dangerous drug across international borders. Like cocaine, even the smallest trace rings alarm bells now the world has turned its back on British beef. Egypt won't let in British leather, Taiwanese consumers worry about British milk powder and Danish shoppers are wondering what the British put in wine gums. U.S. troops serving in Europe are getting their hamburger meat from back home. Jordan has banned British chocolate bars.

3/28/96 AMMAN - Jordan banned imports of British dairy products after Britain said it had found a likely link between mad cow disease, and its deadly human equivalent, Creutzfeldt-Jakob disease. "After the suspension decision, our inspectors went around major supermarkets, importer warehouses and shops to collect and impound all British and Irish-made chocolate, cheese and dairy products and derivatives in circulation," a government official stated.

3/28/96 WASHINGTON - The Food and Drug Administration said it would consider banning the feeding of cattle and sheep remains to cattle because of the scare over "mad cow" disease. Spokesman Lawrence Bachorik said the FDA would decide in the next 10-14 days whether to issue regulations based on an August 1994 proposal to ban the use of goats and certain parts of sheep in animal feeds. When asked whether the final rules would include a ban on the use of cattle parts, Bachorik said it might. It's definitely something we would look at. A final rule could be published within three months, he said. A spokesman for the National Cattlemen/s Beef Association said cattle producers would support whatever decision the FDA came to, provided it was based on sound science. "If the FDA has the scientific basis for such a ban, we would support their action," said animal health expert Gary Weber.

Commenting on this I would say that this is a National Public Health emergency and that these feeding practices should be prohibited at once, otherwise many lives will be lost as occurring in Britain. As a Epidemiologist I would ask what scientific proof do they want? We already have a statistically and epidemiological relationship. What else is needed. Look at what is happening in Britain.

3/28/96 LONDON - Plans to slaughter tens of thousands of British cattle because of the scare over mad cow disease would face huge practical problems, farming sources said today. Industry sources said there were hardly any of the incinerators needed to reach the high temperatures essential to destroy the infective agents of the disease. Britain has only 10 incinerator plants, which have an annual capacity of 50,000 cattle a year but are already busy destroying 300 animals, with the disease, each week. Older cattle are most likely to have the disease, and the National Farmers Union proposed killing 15,000 older cattle a week. A more radical option is to slaughter all cattle in herds that have been touched by BSE, a total of about two million head, and a total cost of up to six billion pounds.

3/29/96 TURIN, Italy - British farmers called for urgent extra measures, including the mass incineration of cattle, to tackle the crisis over mad cow disease and restore consumer confidence in beef. "We want suspect British cattle taken completely off the market and incinerated," said Martin Haworth, head of international affairs of the National Farmers' Union. He said British farm minister Douglas Hogg's announcement on banning the sale of beef, from newly-slaughtered cows, over 30 months old was a first step but was not enough.

3/29/96 LONDON - A Cambodian newspaper suggested that Britain send cattle to Cambodia to detonate landmines left over from decades of regional war. "The English have 11 million mad cows and Cambodia has roughly the same number of equally mad land mines.

British farmers facing the worse crisis to hit their industry in decades want quick, drastic action. "We want suspect British cattle taken completely off the market and incinerated," Martin Haworth, head of the international affairs department of Britain's National Farmers' Union, told a news conference in Turin.

3/29/96 BUENOS AIRES, Argentina - Argentina has agreed to support the European Union in the World Trade Organization in its battle with the United States over the European Union's ban on hormones in beef, German Farm Minister Jochen Borchert said. "We agreed that it is first of all necessary to fight against BSE, but second to keep the ban on hormones and cattle fattening."

3/29/96 LONDON - British carnivores, gripped with panic over mad cow disease, are deserting roast beef for crocodile and ostrich steaks. The meat counter at the luxury London departments store Harrods is doing a brisk trade in emu and kangaroo steaks, ostrich and alligator fillets. The Vegetarian Society, which estimates that one in five Britons is vegetarian, has found its hotline constantly blocked with a stream of anxious callers. It is careful not to crow about the disease. "It is very difficult to be gleeful about the mass slaughter of animals and the loss of human life," said spokeswoman Samantha Calvert. "But this has made the public realize what hidden nasties go into their food. We are pleased people realize the price we have to pay for meat eating."

3/29/96 BRUSSELS - British farmers, have proposed a massive slaughter campaign aimed at restoring the public's appetite for the meat. It is estimated 850,000 animals would be killed in the first year with 750,000 a year thereafter for an unspecified duration. Due to environmental concerns the carcasses would have to be disposed of by incineration. However, Britain has only 10 such incinerators and they are already running at capacity burning 1,000 older cows and bulls each week because of infection with bovine spongiform encephalopathy.

3/29/95 CANBERRA, Australia - Australia joined the long list of countries closing their doors to all products linked to British beef in the midst of the mad cow scare. The banned products included soups, canned foods, stock cubes and sauces and would take effect immediately with stores around the country ordered to remove these products from their shelves. Members of the public with such foods in their cupboards were advised to put them aside.

3/30/96 ALEXANDRIA - Egypt loosened an import ban impose on European beef and cattle and said it would allow in 5,200 Irish cattle stranded in ships, for a week, because of a mad cow disease scare.

3/30/96 PARIS - The French government has launched a campaign to soothe consumers' fears by putting special labels on French beef. But fears persisted. A militant French farm union threatened to stage commando-style raids on British trucks and set fire to any beef being smuggled into France. French farmers torched truckloads of British sheep during a summer of violence in 1990 caused by cuts in farm subsidies.

3/30/96 BERN, Switzerland - Two cases of mad cow disease have been reported in Switzerland, pushing the number recorded so far this year to 20, the Federal Veterinary Office said today. In 1995, 68 cases of mad cow disease were discovered in Switzerland, the second highest number in Europe after Britain.

3/30/96 BRUSSELS - European Union officials are working on plans ranging from selective slaughter to new animal feed rules. European Union sources said the package under discussion included new rules on how to carve up carcasses, a ban on selling for human consumption meat from cattle over 30 months old, and rules forcing animal remains destined for recycling to be cooked at higher temperatures than currently use. Part of the blame for the prevalence in England of mad cow disease, they said, was the fact that during the first oil crisis in the early 1970's offal cooking temperatures had been reduced to save money. They had never been raised again. The National Farmers Union of England and Wales has called for killing 85,000 cattle in the first year followed by three-quarters of a million cattle a year thereafter. But incinerators in Britain can only cope with 50,000 carcasses a year. The European Union sources said this capacity problem could be coped with by licensing premises to kill the cattle and bury them in lime pits.

3/31/96 CAIRO - Police in the Egyptian port city of Alexandria said they had arrested a man who stabbed his wife for refusing to cook imported meat because she was scared it was infected with "mad cow" disease. The woman is in the hospital in critical condition and her husband has been detained for interrogation, police said.

3/31/96 LONDON - Tony Blair, leader of the opposition Labor party said ministers had been "woefully incompetent" in their handling of the crisis. "The government insults the intelligence of people by trying to blame what has happened on the media, the opposition, the consumer or anyone else," Blair told the BBC.

3/31/96 LONDON - Governments must make judgments and I believe the judgment is to take out those animals at the end of the food chain which were exposed to the active BSE agent in the years 1984-89," said David Naish, president of the powerful National Farmers' Union. "It will require money because there is a cashflow problem in the industry, quite apart from the cost of taking out the old animals."

4/1/96 PLOURAC'H, France - French health officials on Monday began destroying a 124 -strong herd of cattle in the Brittany village of Plourac'h after one animal was found to have mad cow disease. The destruction, which began at dawn under strong police guard was expected to be completed by midday, officials said. The bodies will be incinerated in nearby Nantes.

4/1/96 GENEVA - A World Health Organization met for the two-day crisis meeting in Geneva, behind close-doors sessions, and clamped a news blackout until after the meeting.

4/1/96 TAIWAN - It was announced that a consignment of blood serum imported from the United States was contaminated with Creutzfeldt-Jakob Disease. One of the U.S. donors, that contributed to a 1995 consignment of some 3,000 shots of albumin serum injected into Taiwanese patients, was infected with CJD.

4/1/96 TOKYO - Food retailers and wholesalers in Japan have been told to show the origin of imported beef in an attempt to ease concerns over mad cow disease, the Agriculture Ministry said it will mean shops having to display stickers stating the origin of imported beef.

4/2/96 NEW DELHI - A Hindu group in India offered to shelter British cows threatened with slaughter because of mad cow disease, but denied it planned to ship 12 million of them to sanctuary in India. The radical Vishwa Hindu Parishad (World

Hindu Council) said that they had told representatives in London to build a shelter for "homeless cows" and cows with the disease. "We have given directions to our unit in London that they should administer medical aid to the cows that have gone mad and to homeless cows, and build a shelter for them," a spokesman said. "A special place will be allocated after discussions with the government where we will look after the cows," the spokesman said. "If people kill our helpless cows so that they do not die by eating beef, it is not morally correct." Last week VHP officials said Britain deserved to have its $6 billion beef farming collapse overnight because it raised cows solely for slaughter. "This is God's way of teaching them a lesson," VHP leader Ashok Singhal said. God has granted them wisdom and they will eventually stop eating beef this way." He did not say how many cows VHP might shelter.

4/2/96 BRUSSELS - The European Cosmetic, Toiletry and perfumery Association said the cosmetic industry had not called for a withdrawal of cosmetic products containing bovine tissue. It said it had agreed to fully reassure consumers that its members do not use biological extracts of bovine tissue with the highest risk potential (brain, eye and central nervous system).

4/2/96 BRATISLAVIA - Slovakia today banned all imports of beef and beef products from Britain and other countries where mad cow disease has appeared. This is to guarantee that infected animals, groceries and animal feed from the countries with mad cow disease will not get into our stocks, Agriculture Minister Peter Baco said.

4/2/96 LISBON - Portugal is preparing an emergency plan to tackle mad cow disease. The plan aims to detect possible focuses of infection and to eliminate them, Prime Minister Antonio Guterres told reporters during a visit to northern Portugal where most of the country's 36 cases of mad cow disease had been identified.

4/2/96 GENEVA - Hiroshi Nakajima, WHO director-general said in an opening speech distributed by the 190-member agency, "Cattle products, such as meat and milk, are widely consumed and important sources of protein in many countries. Therefore the safety of these products is a global nutritional security issue as well as one of major economic importance." Among those taking part is James Ironside of the National Creutzfeldt-Jakob Surveillance Unit at Western General Hospital in Edinburgh, Scotland, who examined the brains of the victims of the new degenerative disease which causes dementia and loss of neuromuscular control. Others are from Australia, Austria, Canada, France, Germany Ireland, Italy, Japan, Russia, Switzerland and the United States.

4/2/96 LUXEMBOURG - The British delegation was not able to convince other members of the European Union that its plan to deal with the eradication of the so-called mad cow disease was sufficient to restore confidence in the safety of British beef. British Agriculture Minister Douglas Hogg pledged that Britain would go well beyond scientific recommendations in order to convince consumers that British beef is safe to eat. He said a program would be launched to prevent all cows older than 30 months from ever entering the food chain, even if they continued to work as dairy cows. He said a program would involve the slaughter and incineration of some 15,000 cows per week for up to six years—for a maximum total of 4.6 million cattle—at an estimated cost of as much as $450 million. Another estimated $300 million would be spent on eliminating younger cows in herds with incidence of BSE. However, the British program did not go as far as some countries would like. They proposed slaughtering all herds with even one case of BSE.

4/2/96 London - London has agreed to imposing stronger controls on registering and tracking British beef and to implement a fail-safe BSE-sanitizing system for bone and animal feed. The indiscriminate use of cow and sheep brains and spinal columns for cattle feed was considered to have magnified the British BSE problem well beyond the banning of the practice in 1989.

4/3/96  NAIROBI - Kenya has warned all its ports against letting through imported meat and meat products and told public health officers to guard against businessmen who may import them from Britain. Chief Public Health Officer Kefa Ajode warned Kenya might become a dumping ground for meat products infected with bovine spongiform encephalopathy. Be aware of unscrupulous businessmen trying to import cheap meat, and their products, from the United Kingdom, to make quick money from unsuspecting Kenyans.  Libya announced it was banning imports of beef, milk and beef by-products from Britain and some other European countries.

4/3/96 LONDON - The European Union refused to lift a ban on Britain's beef and cattle exports.  Britain, which has insisted its beef is safe to eat, denounced the continued ban and said it was urgently examining whether it was legal.  "That ban is not justified.  It is not based on sound scientific analysis.  It is disproportionate.  It should be removed."  Agriculture Minister Douglas Hogg told parliament. In Belgium, farmers herded cattle into a busy Brussels street under a banner stating "The world is mad, our cows are not."

4/3/96 LUXEMBOURG - The following are among the measures agreed by European Union farm ministers.  British cattle over the age of 30 months, when slaughtered, cannot enter the food chain.  Carcasses must be destroyed.  Specified offal, as defined by Britain in a March plan to combat BSE, must be removed from both the human and animal food chain.  The cost of destroying cattle and their remains will be the responsibility of the British government.  The European Union will contribute 70 percent of the cost of the compensation for the animals themselves. Britain will pay 30 percent.

4/3/96 WASHINGTON DC - The FDA  said it has no plans to ban cattle-derived products from diet supplements or cosmetics despite the scare over "mad cow" disease in Britain. The agency asked makers of dietary supplements in 1992 not to use cattle products from countries where BSE was present but the voluntary ban will not be made official, spokesman Arthur Whitmore said. Raw cattle organs and glands are used in nutritional supplements and as a natural source of hormones. Animal parts are also rendered to make tallow used in soap and cosmetics. Many products contain parts from cows. Processed cow fats are sometimes used to make cookies and salty snacks taste rich. They make lipsticks glide smoothly. Cow proteins show up in shampoo. And gelatin which comes from cattle hide and bones, is also used for capsules that encase drugs capsules. It is also used in candy, desserts, ice cream and many other foods. While there was no indication that there was any product in the United States contaminated with BSE, Whitmore said, its presence in dietary supplements was possible.

4\4\96 ATLANTA - The Centers for Disease Control and Prevention said it has begun tracking a human brain disorder believed to be linked to mad cow disease. The federal health agency announced immediate measures to examine cases of Creutzfeldt - Jakob Disease in four states that already have advanced health surveillance systems in place. Noting that there are four strains of the disease, the CDC said it wants to make sure an unusual strain found recently in Britain is not present in the United States.

4/4/96 AUSTIN - Texas Agriculture Commissioner Rick Perry criticized the U.S. media for stoking fears among domestic beef consumers. "We've got everyone from radio disc jockeys to NBC's Dateline inferring that eating beef exposes you to this disease." Perry said, offering reporters slices of the thinly sliced, freshly smoked brisket.

4/4/96 LONDON - Cats and dogs are better protected than humans from the mad cow disease, Andrew Mackin a veterinary expert said and that it would be safer to eat a can of dog food than a beefburger in summer of 1989. Farmers in Britain told the government it will have to shoot them first if it wants to slaughter whole herds.

4/4/96 TURKEY - Turkey's agriculture ministry lifted a ban on leather imports from certain European countries but said British cow hides would remain banned as a precaution against mad cow disease. The ministry banned all animal product imports from Britain, Ireland, Switzerland, Portugal and France on March 27, 1996 in view of concern about the disease.

4/4/96 PARIS - France said it had registered a case of the fatal human brain illness Creutzfeldt-Jakob Disease (CJD) similar to British cases but did not know if it was linked to mad cow disease. Chief health officer Jean-Francois Girard told a news conference that the case was comparable to those recorded in Britain. Should we panic? Of course not, we cannot say anything more than we are in an uncertain situation, he added. Girard said the French case concerned a 26-year-old man who died last January in Lyon. Anatomical data showed it was similar to the 10 British cases.

4/5/96 EDINBURGH - Gerald Collee of the University of Edinburgh said in a letter to the editor of Lancet, "At some time in the mid 1980s or the early 1990, many foods contain bovine brain and other offal such as spinal cord and parts of the intestine and used in sausage and other ground beef products for years. A microbiologist Steve Dealler said as many as one million people in Britain could develop CJD.

4/5/96 LONDON - In the Lancet medical journal on April 5, 1996 Dr. Robert Will said 10 new cases were very unusual because the victims were young, between 19 and 41. Usually CJD with an incubation period of up to 30 years, usually affects people over 60. Only one person under the age of 30 had died of CJD in Britain between 1970 and 1994. Five died in 1995 and 1996. Dr. Will said the cases were found by checking everyone in Britain with suspected CJD. The cases all had the spongy holes characteristic of such diseases, including BSE, and a waxy buildup known as plaque which is also seen in Alzheimer's, another form of dementia. This plaque was made up of proteins known as prions and in a form resembling those found in kuru, a brain disease that use to kill cannibals in Papua-New Guinea who ritualistically ate human brains. Prions somehow mutate to cause the disease. This unusual feature was not seen in any of the other 175 random CJD cases investigated. Similar lesions have been seen in cases of scrapie. All nine cases were reported to have eaten beef or beef products in the last 10 year, but none was reported to have eaten brain. The Lancet criticized the government reaction to the report, accusing ministers of defending the beef industry at the expense of public health. In the editorial of the Lancet it said the government seemed to hear only what it wanted to hear. When Dr. Robert Will said "I believe this is a new phenomenon, there is reason for major concern, the remark was unheeded." It called for a new separate government agency to handle such issues, a independent agency that reports to the public, not the policy makers.

4/6/96 VERONA, Italy - A 60-year-old Italian man has died of the fatal human brain illness Creutzfeldt-Jakob Disease. Guiseppe Fettari, head of neurology, at a Verona hospital , said "Nobody would have noticed this case if the death had come about just one month ago."

4/6/96 STRASBOURG, France - France, the first country in the Union to ban British beef exports, said earlier this week it will slaughter about 70,000 British born veal calves impounded at the height of the crisis but at no faster pace than they would have been killed anyway.

4/7/96 LONDON - Britain's Hindu community joined in prayer Sunday for the millions of cattle expected to be slaughtered to prevent any risk of mad cow disease spreading to people. Religious leaders led prayers among Britain's estimated 140,000 Hindus for the doomed herds. The cow is sacred to Hindus, who try to observe a vegetarian diet.

4/9/96 LYON, France - French doctors said they had no new information on how a case of the fatal human Creutzfeldt -

Jakob Disease registered in Lyon, and identical to British cases, had been transmitted. The Lyon hospital authority said after local brain surgeons traveled to Britain to exchange information that the British unit monitoring CJD cases had confirmed the French case was "absolutely similar" to British cases.

4/9/96 SAN FRANCISCO - A California woman had died of Creutzfeldt -Jakob disease, but there is no reason to suspect a link to "mad cow" disease which had caused a scare in Britain, officials said. Carol Vanetti, 58, died of CJD at St. Joseph's in Stockton, California, said hospital spokesman Jim Shebl. Doctors diagnosed the incurable, brain-destroying illness after Vanetti was admitted to the hospital last month following a fall, he said. Doctors do not know how Vanetti, a Stockton resident, contracted the disease, which victims can carry for up to 30 years before showing symptoms, he said.

In relation to the foregoing news item, I was at Hazard canyon on the beach near Morro Bay, California talking to two graduates of Cal Poly, in Agriculture Business Economics, who are involved now in providing feed for cows. One stated he was eating a Hamburger, driving in Stockton, California when he heard the announcement on the radio of Carol Vanetti dying of CJD. He had to lay his burger down and not eat anymore of it. The two Cal Poly graduates stated they were doing all they could that cows be fed high quality alfalfa hay and other protein sources from plants rather than dead animals to be fed to Beef and Dairy cows. Learning their intentions made my day!

4/10/96 BRUSSELS - Senior European Union veterinary officials eased a ban on British exports of cattle and meat products. The experts said that gelatin and tallow were safe if certain (manufacturing) processes are followed. Gelatin, a thickening agent widely used in food, including yogurt, jellies and sweets, and tallow, one of the main ingredients in bar soaps, are both obtained from cattle carcasses. The committee

95

is expected to clarify whether the ban covers finished medicinal, cosmetic and pharmaceutical products or only British beef ingredients in those products.

4/10/96 LISBON - A Portuguese medical official said the human equivalent of mad cow disease could be contracted from certain medicines containing cattle products and called for them to be banned. "We do not wish to cause alarm, but we are concerned that the disease is much more likely to be spread by using these medicines than by eating beef." Said Carols Ribeiro, President of the Portuguese Medical Association. He said the Portuguese Medical Association would press for the ban on some 30 medicines during the meeting with Health Minister Maria de Belem Roseira. Doctors said the ban should cover medicines containing cattle offal, which are used to treat obesity in humans. The Portuguese Medical Association said it also wanted a ban on cattle tripe, brains and gizzards which are popular in Portugal. The Agriculture Ministry has said the Portuguese can eat beef without fear of mad cow disease but should avoid consuming brain or cattle bone marrow.

4/10/96 BEIRUT - Lebanon said it had banned imports of cattle and meat and related products from Britain and Ireland to calm consumers after the mad cow disease scare. Agriculture Minister Shawki Fakhoury said the ban covered cows, sheep and goats, their meat, meat or bone flour used in animal fodder, canned meat or other produce, bull semen, frozen sperm or cattle embryos from Britain and Ireland.

4/10/96 BRUSSELS, Belgium - European Union officials dashed British hopes of ending the mad cow crisis with a decision to leave a ban on beef exports in place and unchanged. "The decision is bitterly disappointing, particularly following the World Health Organization's endorsement of the safety of British beef products. The UK will fight on until the ban is lifted ," Britain's Ministry of Agriculture said in a statement issued in London.

4/10/96 BUENOS AIRES, Argentina - Argentina intends to use the 11th annual regional congress of the International Meat Secretariat to further polish its image as a growing provider of natural, free range grass-fed beef free of both BSE and the hormones that lurk in the steaks of some competing exporters like the United States.

4/10/96 PARK RIDGE, Ill. - The American Farm Bureau Federation urged livestock and government officials to locate and destroy all imported British cattle found on U.S. farms. Authorities are searching for 35 of these animals they cannot locate. Farm Bureau President Dean Kleckner said U.S. livestock producers are taking strong action to restore consumer confidence in the U.S. beef supply.

4/10/96 LONDON - Japanese scientist, Shigeru Katamine, a bacteriologist at the Nagasake School of Medicine, published in the science journal Nature stated evidence that the proteins, known as prions, have a role in such diseases as CJD. In the mad cow disease they seem to mutate, causing the typical spongelike holes in the brain. This also apparently happens in CJD. They said it could be the loss of normal prion protein that causes the damage in disease like CJD and BSE. This would mean that prions are important to brain functions and it is the mutation that kills off normal proteins rather than the prion itself that is dangerous.

4/10/96 WASHINGTON - U.S. veterinary officials said they had destroyed the first 10 out of 113 British cattle in the United States in an effort to prevent "mad cow" disease from entering the country. The cattle, from South Dakota, were incinerated this week and their brains sent for examination to the national veterinary laboratory in Ames, Iowa. There were still 29 British cattle in Alabama, 1 in Arkansas, 1 in Georgia, 2 in Iowa, 2 in Idaho, 3 in Illinois, and 1 each in Kentucky, Louisiana, Minnesota, Mississippi, Montana and New Hampshire, officials said. There were also 13 in New York, 5 in Oklahoma, 4 in Pennsylvania, 3 in Tennessee, 22 in Texas, 8 in

Vermont, 1 in Wisconsin and 3 in West Virginia.

4/10/96 LONDON - Mark Robinson of the Animal Disease Research Unit in Pullman, Wash. Told New Scientist magazine that the U.S. Department of Agriculture had been trying to give cows BSE since 1990. At a laboratory in Ames, Iowa, they injected 18 calves with brain tissues from sheep that had scrapie. The cows got sick, but it wasn't BSE. Robinson said "The pathology in the brain did not resemble BSE at all," he told New Scientist.

Britain's Agriculture Ministry resisted saying people could get the human form of the disease, Creutzfeldt - Jakob Disease, from eating infected beef for 10 years. They said CJD had never been linked to scrapie and people had been eating sheep and sheep's brains for centuries. The government had to change its line last month when scientists said they had identified a new strain of CJD, one that could be linked to eating beef.

Robert Rohwer, and expert on spongiform encephalopathy at the Veterans Affairs Medical Center in Baltimore, said the U.S. research could make British government advisers think hard. "If it is not scrapie in cows, that blows the whole basis of the public health policy out of the window." Rohwer said he could not understand why British scientists were not conducting similar experiments. British government veterinarians say they do not need to give sheep scrapie to cows in order to confirm or negate the theory, but that it is obvious cattle get BSE from sheep remains. Rohwer told the magazine he thought BSE was a new disease that arose in British cows and pointed out that cattle carcasses were also ground up into the cows' food. The infectious agent would have been repeatedly recycled in the cows through their food, eventually causing the epidemic.

4/11/96 LONDON - Fears that mad cow disease might be spread to people who eat beef have led to a further alarm—that pregnant women might pass the deadly human counterpart to their babies said Dr. Sheila Gore, a Biostatistics researcher at the British government's Medical Research Council told New Scientist magazine. The slow onset of the disease means that no one knows how many people, or how many young women, may be carrying it. "For the first time we are seeing cases of CJD among women still in their childbearing years. Because this has never happened before we have no idea of the risk of maternal infection. There is a serious need to quantify this." Some scientists think this is evidence that cows pass it to their calves. To find out, John Wilesmith of the Government's Central Veterinary Laboratory is following the lives of 300 calves born to BSE - infected cows in 1988 and 1989 and another 300 born to non-infected cows. At least 45 animals in the experiment have already died from BSE, according to the New Scientist report.

4\11\96 AALTEN, Netherlands - The Netherlands began to slaughter 64,000 imported British calves because of fears of mad cow disease. The planned three-stage cull is expected to take five to six weeks and involves killing the animals, crushing their bodies and then burning them at separate locations and is expected to take five or six weeks.

4/11/96 LOS ANGELES - Dr. Michael Harrington of California Institute of Technology in suburban Pasadena said that he had developed a simple test to diagnose "mad cow" disease that could possibly be used to prevent the wholesale slaughter of British cattle. He said, that the test had proved accurate in humans, cows and other animals. Harrington, is working with a team of scientists at the National Institutes of Health in Bethesda, Md., said he expected to submit his paper on the 4/12/96 to the New England Journal of Medicine. Using the new test, a handful of technicians will be able to test an estimated 2,000 cows a month, giving it widespread application. Harrington said in the thousands of human cases he has examined using both the old test and the new test, only three diagnoses have been found to be inaccurate.

4/11/96 ATLANTA - The number of cases of a rare human brain disorder possibly linked to mad cow disease in Britain has remained stable in the United States since 1979, federal health officials said. The U.S. Centers for Disease Control and Prevention (CDC) remained constant at approximately one case per million persons between 1979- and 1993, the latest year for which figures are available. There is no indication that cases of CJD already reported in the U.S. involve the new variant, but investigators will review past cases as part of a more aggressive surveillance effort. "We'll be able to more specifically look and see if this new variant has, in fact, appeared in this country," Howard said. "We really want to hone in on exactly how many cases there are and take a closer look at the cases that are occurring."

4/12/96 BONN Germany - Many Germans see the current mad cow disease scare as a typical example of what happens when humans "pervert" nature, in this case by feeding grass-eating cattle with animal remains.

4/12/96 WASHINGTON - British opposition leader Tony Blair, buoyed by a crushing victory in a by-election at home, crowned a successful United States visit with talks at the White House with President Clinton. Clinton and Blair, tapped as the next British prime minister, discussed Bosnia, trade and protectionism and ways of restoring market confidence after the scare about "mad cow" disease that has hit British beef exports.

4/12/96 LISBON - Portugal's attorney-general's office said it is looking into allegations by top government veterinarians that between 1990 and 1993 the government covered up the extent of mad cow disease in the country. The attorney-general's office said it was studying whether to recommend a full-scale inquiry into the allegations. The move came after two veterinarians told a parliamentary committee that they were silenced by then-Agriculture Minister Arlindo Cunha and their reports into the disease covered up.

The allegations were made by Alexandre Galo, a researcher at the Lisbon Veterinary Laboratory, and Azevedo

Ramos, former head of the National Veterinary Laboratory, and Azevedo Ramos, former head of the National Veterinary Research Laboratory, both of whom have spent time in Britain studying bovine spongiform encephalopathy, commonly known as mad cow disease. Galo said the government measures to combat mad cow disease announced earlier this month should have been taken in 1990. "Measures were taken by my superiors to suppress my findings. My report six years ago said the disease existed here, Galo said on Lisbon radio TSF. Galo's allegations were backed by Socialist lawmaker Antonio Campos who called for measures against mad cow disease six years ago. "There has been scientific censorship and lies on the part of the previous Social Democrat government. I myself was denied access to analyses in 1990. "The government surrendered to pressures from lobby groups instead of caring about the consumer," Campos said. Health ministry figures published this month revealed that 36 people have died in Portugal since 1980 of Creutzfeld-Jakob disease, the human form of mad cow disease.

4/13/96 LONDON - Every time Paul Andrews forgets something, he wonders whether his brain is slowly turning into a sponge. It is a real fear. Andrews believes he is at risk of developing the brain-rotting Creutzfeldt-Jakob Disease (CJD) after treatment to help him reach a normal height as a teenager. "You have the fear every day," said Andrews, a 30-year-old student teacher. "The initial symptoms that you get are exactly like everybody gets when they are tired—you get dizzy, you forget things. I'm always forgetting things, all the bloody time."

He is one of 1,900 Britons given Human Growth Hormone (HGH) to boost their stunted height as children. The hormone was taken from the pituitary glands of corpses. Sixteen British children given the treatment between 1958 and 1985 have died of CJD and one is suffering from it. A lawsuit opening in London's High Court on Tuesday alleges they contracted CJD as a result of the treatment.

Eight families are suing the Health Department and the government-funded Medical Research Council in a case sure to attract attention in the midst of a scare over mad cow disease. With Andrews, from the ages of 11 to 17, he was given three hormone injections a week. For him it did work—he grew a foot to five feet five inches.

Lawyer David Body said "This is a grim business. I don't think anyone can think of a worse way to die than CJD." Parents of the dead children say they were never told the HGH was being taken from corpses. They say more precautions should have been taken over a transplant of human material. "The risk involved was pointed out to the Medical Research Council by agricultural scientists who had an interest in scrapie and who told them there was a risk," Body said.

4/13/96 PARIS - Luc Montagnier, French discoverer of the HIV virus that causes AIDS, said that an AIDS-style pandemic of mad cow disease could not be ruled out but was not likely at the moment. Asked about the likelihood of and AIDS-style pandemic of mad cow disease, Montagnier said: "It's a catastrophe-scenario which cannot be ruled out, but it is not the most likely now. We will know more in a year's time."

Montagnier accused politicians of under-estimating public health dangers. "Our way of life, medical and industrial advances lead in a way to the selection of our future enemies which are stronger agents. "Intensive farming for example stuffs calves, cows and pigs with antibiotics, hormones ... When I see that, I am 100 percent ecologist."

4/14/96 CULLMAN, Alabama - A standoff continued between a north Alabama rancher and state officials over 29 head of British Charolais cows the state wants to purchase and destroy. Agriculture officials contend the planned destruction of the cows is in response to an epidemic of mad cow disease currently infecting British herds. The state wants to kill Forrest Ingram's 29 cows even though the herd has tested negative for the disease in each of the last four years. Ingram's price is $20,000 per head. The average price for American-bred cattle in the region is less than $2,000. Elaine Clayton a Cullman County resident said "Money is not that important to me. My family's health would be my number one concern."

4/14/96 LONDON - Britain's farmers, outraged after the European Union farm commissioner said he thought British beef was safe to eat, called on for a quick end to the EU's ban on beef exports. Commissioner Franz Fischler told Reuters in an interview in Austria that he personally would have no worries about eating British beef despite a scare over mad cow disease. He said a global ban on British beef was aimed at protecting the European beef market. His comments enraged Britons who fear a major industry could be destroyed. "It is ironic that he (Fischler) will eat our beef but won't allow us to export it so that others can eat and enjoy it, a spokesman at Britain's Ministry of Agriculture said. "This is an absolutely astonishing situation. Here is the man who has made Britain a scapegoat and is victimizing the British farmer and the British taxpayer now conceding that all this was done just for the convenience of Europe," Conservative Sir Gerard Vaughan said.

4/15/96 ATHENS - If British livestock breeders had read the works of ancient Greek writers and mythology, they might have averted an outbreak of the fatal mad cow disease , the state-owned Athens News Agency (ANA) suggested yesterday. The report came amid heightened European Union action to eradicate the brain-racking malady, four weeks after British authorities acknowledged its deadly effects on human consumers. The newspaper said British livestock breeders might have prevented the deadly disease had they read the tragedy of Glaucos by the ancient Greek writer Aeschylus.

"The ancient Greek tragedy's moral lesson is that going against nature by feeding flesh to herbivorous animals leads to destruction and havoc," citing Greek intellectuals. "It is not that the ancient Greek mythological gods awoke from centuries of sleep to punish British livestock breeders, but rather it was nature, which does not forgive such transgressions."

Aeschylus' tragedy, written in the 5$^{th}$ century B.C., is about the mythological hero Glaucos, who fed human flesh to his prize stable of mares to make them more ferocious in battle. But Glaucos' action enraged the gods, who cursed his mares. The tragedy ends with the horses going mad and devouring Glaucos.

"Then it was mad horses, today it is mad cows. The moral precept, however, has remained unaltered throughout the centuries," ANA said. Since the mad cow crisis surfaced in Britain, health officials in Athens have confiscated over 60 tons of British beef products and urged panic-stricken Greek consumers to opt for domestic beef.

4/16/96 RABAT - Morocco has banned beef imports from Britain, Ireland and Switzerland, the official news agency MAP reported today. The ban applies to animal produce, both natural and industrial, derived from beef.

4/16/96 PARIS - France said it would destroy 70,000 British-born veal calves to prevent their meat from being sold because of fears it may be infected with mad cow disease. "These British-born calves that we have previously quarantined will now be destroyed so they cannot be sold," French farm minister Philippe Vasseur told parliament. In a bid to prop up consumer confidence, France has begun labeling its beef with "French meat" stickers, drawing complaints from Belgian farmers that their exports had been harmed.

4/16/96 LONDON - Official sources said the government had not ruled out taking the Brussels authorities to the European Union Court of Justice. The National Farmers' Union (NFU) said it was considering action following remarks by EU Agricultural Commissioner Franz Fischler that he personally thought it was safe to eat British beef. The ban, he said, was needed to prevent a collapse of the whole European beef market.

"Mr. Fischler's remarks would appear to contradict the Commission's imposition of the ban on the grounds of protecting public health," NFU president Sir David Naish told reporters. British vets have said they will oppose a mass cull, arguing that is it neither morally nor scientifically justified. Fischler also made clear he believed that BSE was purely a British phenomenon.  It was also clear, he said, that BSE in Britain was linked to feed including ground-up animal parts, and to abuse of regulations designed to halt the spread of the disease. Even though it had been illegal in Britain since 1990 to feed animal meal to grazing animals like cows, this had not been sufficiently adhered to, Fischler said.  Some farmers had obviously bought pig feed and fed it to cows, he added.  Calling for worldwide standards for feed, Fischler said one point had to be stuck to,  meat must not be fed to herbivores.

4/16/96   WASHINGTON - U.S. talk show hosts Oprah Winfrey took on the beef industry saying she would stop eating hamburgers because of fears over mad cow disease.  Winfrey said on her show she was shocked after a guest said meat and bone meal made from cattle was routinely fed to other cattle to boost their meat and milk production.  "It has just stopped me cold from eating another burger," Winfrey said.

Other guests on ABC's Oprah Winfrey Show included Briton Beryl Rimmer, who said her granddaughter contracted CJD from eating beef.  American Linda Marker said her mother-in-law died recently of CJD after eating beef in Britain in 1986.

"Every possible effort has been taken to make sure (a BSE outbreak) never happens here," said Weber, an animal health expert at the National Cattlemen's Beef Association.

4/16/96  LONDON - Human growth hormone prepared at a single British laboratory was probably responsible for infecting 17 children with the brain-wasting Creutzfeldt-Jakob Disease (CJD) lawyer Robert Owen said in opening arguments at the High Court trial, expected to last six weeks.

4/17/96  BRUSSELS - France accused Britain of going back on a promise to slaughter cattle at risk from mad cow disease on a massive scale and also criticized its plan to mount a legal challenge to the European Union ban on British beef exports. British Farm Minister Douglas Hogg said the government was not planning mass slaughter of its beef herds, apparently contradicting an undertaking given to EU farm ministers at an emergency meeting in Luxembourg two weeks ago. Hogg said that slaughtering a large proportion of the 11 million head of British cattle was unrealistic. He also ruled out slaughtering whole herds where BSE outbreaks have occurred, as some other EU countries have done. A British eradication scheme would only be implemented if the EU ban was lifted, he added.

4/17/96 LONDON - Scientist told British law makers it was safe to eat beef, but admitted they are not certain what causes mad cow disease and are far from having a reliable test for it. The members of parliament were told millions of people could be infected with CJD, The human form of BSE—bovine spongiform encephalopathy—known as mad cow disease. Dr. Stephen Dealler, a senior registrar at Burnley General Hospital in northern England, said it was impossible to tell how many people would come down with CJD from eating infected beef. "The worst case scenario is in the millions," he told the committee. "I wouldn't disagree at all that this current range of what is possible could happen," said John Pattison, chairman of the Spongiform Encephalopathy Advisory Committee, which advises the government on mad cow, CJD and similar diseases.

"I consider beef products to be safe to eat in the UK for adults," he said. "The advantage of stopping is really rather small at this time." But he would not feed them to children. "There's a statistical advantage in not feeding beef to children that have not been fed beef before."

Dealler, who stopped eating beef in 1988, said it was possible that beef liver, which is still sold and eaten, could contain the infection. "We have been exporting large numbers of infected cattle to Europe. I have almost a greater worry for the risk that has been taken on in France," he added.

4/17/96 LONDON - The prion protein believed by many

scientist to be responsible for mad cow disease and the related human version may also help regulate sleep, researchers reported today. Irene Tobler of the Institute of Pharmacology at the University of Zurich, and colleagues, said mice bred to produce no prion proteins showed sleep disturbances and seemed unable to tell night from day properly.

"We provide evidence that the prion protein may ... be involved in the regulation of sleep and that loss of this function may result in neurodegeneration in one of the prion diseases, fatal familial insomnia," they wrote in the science journal Nature. "In mice devoid of prion protein there is an alteration in both circadian activity rhythms and sleep patterns." Circadian rhythm governs the night to day cycle of the body. Most experts think Bovine Spongiform Encephalopathy (BSE or mad cow disease) is caused by mutated prions, proteins found in the brain. Related diseases like scrapie in sheep and Creutzfeldt-Jakob Disease (CJD), kuru and fatal familial insomnia in humans are also prion related. The diseases are all marked by loss of memory, followed by loss of muscle coordination, weakness, and death.

4/17/96 STRASBOURG, France - Britain headed for a collision with its European Union partners today as the European Commission blamed it for causing the mad cow crisis and France rejected lifting an export ban on its beef. British Farm Minister Douglas Hogg said Britain would slaughter cattle over 30 months old which had reached the end of their productive lives and destroy the carcasses instead of processing them into meat pies, pet food and chemicals.

French Farm Minister Philippe Vasseur flatly rejected removal of the ban, and Italian Prime Minister Lambaerto Dini, representing the EU's presidency, shrugged off the threatened challenge, saying the ban should only be lifted when scientific evidence showed the beef and beef products were safe. "I can give you the formal, solemn and strongest assurance that in the current state of affairs, there is no question of lifting the embargo," Vasseur told the French Parliament.

Ben Gill, Deputy President of the National Farmers' Union of England and Wales, said "I cannot accept that this is a public health issue. The measures that have been taken and are being taken deal with all possible sources of infection," Gill said. " There is no suggestion that this beef is unfit to eat."

The European Commission likewise supported the British view that mass slaughter among Britain's 11 million cattle had never been promised.

4/18/96 PRAGUE - British Prime Minister John Major said it "defies logical belief" that the European Union continues its exports ban on British beef while at the same time saying the meat is safe. "We have the assertion from the EU's agricultural commissioner that he would eat British beef, and British beef is safe, we have the same assertion from EU President Santer that British beef is safe," Major said. "On the back of that, it defies logical belief, the ban continues in the way it does."

4/18/96 LONDON - Medicines manufactured in Britain using animal products are probably not infected with mad cow disease, a British doctor said. Dr. Anne Wickham said she thought such medication because the purification methods used in making drugs and injectable insulin would probably kill off any infection even if it got into the medical supply. "Doctors and patients will need to weigh these unknown and possible non-existent risks against the known risks of discontinuing or changing medication ," she wrote in the British Medical Journal.

European Farm Commissioner Franz Fischler provoked British anger last week by admitting the ban had been imposed to save the European beef market, not for scientific reasons. "The commission has never said British beef was not safe Fischler told the European Parliament.

4/18/96 LONDON - British beef industry representative told parliament it had made mistakes in trying to prevent the spread of mad cow disease. Parliament's health and agriculture committees, meeting jointly to investigate BSE or mad cow disease, was told that spot checks revealed lax procedures at slaughterhouses. But Ashley Bowes, president of the Federation of Fresh Meat Wholesalers, said the guidelines sometimes failed. "Unfortunately, we do our best, but we are not perfect," he told the committee.

In a separate report, a government safety committee told slaughterhouse workers that people might possibly get the human version of mad cow disease from handling infected meat and it re-issued the safety guidelines. If laboratory or slaughterhouse workers could get BSE, it would most likely be from infected material getting into cuts, or being breathed in or swallowed, it said.

4/18/96 CHICAGO - Cattle industry officials condemned a recent Oprah Winfrey show on food safety that included a discussion of bovine spongiform encephalopathy, also know as mad cow disease, and it's suspected link to a fatal human disease. The National Cattlemen's Beef Association said the "irresponsible and biased show," hit U.S. farmers and ranchers. "Your April 16 show is one more example of the irresponsible scare tactics with which much of American television has become identified," John Lacey, president of the NCBA, wrote in a letter to Winfrey. "The show was one of beef-bashing—not a reasonable discussion of BSE and the safety of the American beef supply. You took a complex technical issue and turned it into an hour of unjustified scare-mongering." Lacey said the show gave equal time to vegetarian activist Howard Lyman and cattle industry representative Gary Weber during taping, but later edited out three-fourths of Weber's scientific explanation and rebuttal of Lyman.

Winfrey defended the program and her handling of the issue, and announced she will do another show on the subject because of the furor it has caused. "I am speaking as one consumer for millions of others," Winfrey sad in a prepared statements. "Cows eating cows is alarming. Americans needed and wanted to know that—I certainly did." Later, her staff issued another statement saying, "because last Tuesday's show on the dangerous handling of foods sparked enormous interest from viewers, government organizations and the beef industry, the Oprah Winfrey Show is planning another program to address unanswered questions."

5/4/96 TORONTO - The largest children's hospital in Canada has notified 500 families that their children received blood products from donors now infected with deadly Creutzfeldt-Jakob disease, the hospital said today. The Canadian Red Cross products were used at Toronto's Sick Children's Hospital between 1989 and 1995 and the donors have since contracted the brain-wasting illness.

5/4/96 LONDON - Labour member of parliament Gavin Strang said that in the first three months of this year, two-thirds of cows diagnosed as having BSE were born after feed which included animal products had been banned. He believed some farmers were still giving infected feed to cattle despite a 1989 ban and questioned the need for a massive cull.

5/6/96 PARIS - France has slaughtered 123 cattle to destroy one of two herds where the Agriculture Ministry last week reported a case of mad cow disease, officials said on Monday. The herd, at Orglandes near Cherbourg, was the 17th destroyed in France since bovine spongiform encephalopathy (BSE), which rots the brain of cattle, was first registered in the country in 1991.

5/6/96 OTRANTO, Italy - The European Commission is due to decide on Wednesday whether beef products such as gelatin, tallow, should be exempted from a ban on British beef exports, said EU Farm Commissioner Franz Fischler. Fischler stressed it was very important that Britain enforce a ban on feeding meat and bone meal to cattle, improve disease control measures, especially in the meat rendering industry, implement a scheme to slaughter older animals over 30 months and a scheme to slaughter animals most at risk to BSE.

5/8/96 LONDON - A group of biologists predicted up to

24,000 more cases of mad cow disease in Britain before 1999 unless a widespread culling of herds takes place. The European Union is insisting on major culling before it lifts a global ban on British beef because of mad cow disease.

5/8/96 WASHINGTON - Many researchers believe the British public will soon be afflicted with an outbreak of a human variant of the disease called Creutzfeldt-Jakob disease (CJD). The British cattle appear to have picked up the disease after being fed the brain and spinal cords of sheep, which develop a related brain malady called scrapie. The rest of Europe appears to have escaped the epidemic by moving quickly to stop this practice. And in the United States, no cattle are currently afflicted with BSE, according to the U.S. Department of Agriculture. Infectious proteins called prions are the culprits. When they infiltrate the brain, these prions wrap around similar proteins and bend them to match their own disfigured and dysfunctional state. The build up of these defective prions destroys vast areas of the brain and eventually causes death. Martin Novak of University of Oxford in Britain said its possible humans cannot get CJD from beef. They maybe can only get it from eating brain tissue, no one knows for sure. But over the next several years, there may be a significant increase in CJD cases in the UK. It is likely that cattle can pass BSE to humans. For instance, lions, tigers and other large carnivores in zoos have gotten the disease from eating beef, as well as brain matter.

5/8/96 MILAN - Tens of thousands of Italian farmers marched through Milan to demand government action to overcome an economic crisis caused by mad cow disease and European union quotas on agricultural products. The farmers filled Milan's huge Pizaa del Duomo square for a closing rally. Italian television estimated the crowd at 100,000.

5/9/96 LISBON - Portugal began on Thursday slaughtering 1,200 cattle which were imported from Britain or had contact with the 37 cases of the disease reported in Portugal, will be killed and incinerated at a northern slaughterhouse in a three-day campaign.

5/13/96 RIVERDALE - The Food and Drug Administration will publish a proposal on Tuesday to ban certain types of cattle feed derived from cows, sheep and other animals -- that have been associated with mad-cow disease in Britain. Some high-protein feed supplements are made from animal parts including bones and intestines, which are cooked in a process know as rendering and then pulverized. Britain this year banned meat and bone meal from all animal feeds, not just feeds for cud-chewing animals, a step beyond the proposal by the Food and Drug Administration (FDA). Stephen Sundlof, director of FDA's Center for Veterinary Medicine, said on Monday the rule was needed to lessen the risk of an outbreak of so-called mad cow disease in the United States. The proposal would take the form of an advanced notice of rulemaking published in the Federal Register in which FDA calls for public comments. The agency would publish a more formal proposed rule within six months and a final rule within 12 months, a spokesman for Sundlof said.

Scientists and public interest groups at the meeting expressed dismay that FDA Commissioner David Kessler had failed to order and immediate ban on that type of feeding. "An advanced notice of proposed rulemaking is not the most efficient way to get this done," said Caroline Smith de Waal of the Washington-based Center for Science in the Public Interest. The FDA had promised on March 29 to "expedite" the implementation of the ban. A representative of the nation's feed industry questioned the need for the ban, saying it would cost the feed and rendering industries at least $100 million a year. "At this time, we think it is a radical proposition," said American Feed Industry Association nutrition director Richard Sellers. Sellers said there was no need for the ban in the Unites States because there have been no known cases of mad-cow disease. A spokesman for the National Cattlemen's Beef Association welcomed FDA's action as a means of cutting down the risk of an outbreak of the disease. "Our position is, let's just cease this (feeding) practice right now," said NCBHA animal health expert Gary Weber.

5/13/96 MAINZ, Germany - German authorities slaughtered and then burned an entire herd of cattle on Monday to protect the public from the risks of "mad cow" disease, officials said. The 115-head herd belonged to a farmer in the western town of Rennerod in Rhinland-Palatinate state who had bought 40 cows in 1992 from a breeder in Lower Saxony, local officials in Montabaur said. Montabaur officials said the lower Saxony breeder had bought British cattle and animal meal, which can transmit BSE.

5/14/96 LONDON - The family of a woman who died of the human equivalent of mad cow disease are seeking public funds to sue the British government, their lawyer said on Tuesday. Dutch-born Fonnie van Es died two years ago at the age of 44 of Creutzfeldt-Jakob Disease (CJD), a fatal condition that attacks the brain. Lawyer David Harris said he has seeking access to information available to the government on the subject over the past 10 years. "The government made assertions that the safety of British beef was such that it was possible for the public to continue to eat it." London's High Court is currently hearing a lawsuit on behalf of 17 children who contracted CJD after being treated with Human Growth Hormone taken from the brains of human corpses.

5/15/96 BRUSSELS - European Union veterinary officials examined a proposal on Wednesday to ease the worldwide ban on British beef  products despite German-led opposition and criticism that Britain has not yet done enough to combat mad cow disease. Britain's three gelatin factories and the vast bulk of tallow production already complied with proposed strict high temperature heat processing rules to remove any risk of contamination. Gelatin is a thickening agent widely used in yogurt, sweets and other foodstuffs. Tallow is used in bar soaps.

5/15/96 GLASGOW, Scotland - The human form of "mad cow disease" may be more common than anyone ever thought, experts who have studied the brain-wasting illness said today.  As with many other diseases, doctors might be finding Creutzfeldt-Jakob Disease (CJD) more often because they were now looking for it, said Gareth Roberts, an expert on dementia for SmithKline Beecham Pharmaceuticals.  Roberts told a conference of 2,000 European scientists that it was possible earlier cases of CJD had been missed simply because doctors were not looking for it.  "This disease is hugely variable," he said.  "One wonders whether in this particular situation. . . this is a disease indeed that has been there, and now we are looking, we have found it," agreed Roger Feldman, and epidemiologist at Queen Mary and Westfield College in London.  "If you start looking, you may find things you never knew were there before.  It causes demented behavior with victims becoming steadily more uncoordinated.  They always die, and their brains are found to be shrunken and full of holes.  Roberts said it was easy to mix up CJD with other diseases and, as the only way to diagnose it was by looking at the brain after death, it would be very easy to miss.  In older people it was probably mixed up with Alzheimer's disease, while in younger victims it could look like multiple sclerosis or a severe viral infection. Roberts, an expert on Alzheimer's said victims of familial CJD -- a strain inherited by people with a genetic mutation -- had died in their forties but their brains had looked normal.  Studying brain samples he had kept from 1,000 patients who died of dementia between 1964 and 1990, he found 19 CJD cases.  Only 11 had been properly diagnosed at the time, which meant that 40 percent of the cases had gone undetected.  "They were usually mixed up with Alzheimer's" he said.  "I never thought to look at younger people," he added later at a news conference.  He said scientists around the world should be checking to see if they had misdiagnosed cases. But all three scientists agreed it was very possible that people got CJD from eating infected beef.  Roberts said it was also possible some people had been getting it all along from food, although much more work would have to be done to prove this.  Sheep have had scrapie, their own version of the disease, for 200 years, but scientists say people cannot catch scrapie from sheep.

5/22/96 LONDON - Britain went on the offensive against Europe today setting up a crisis committee under Prime Minister John Major to coordinate its new strategy of paralyzing European business until a beef export ban is lifted. Majors patience finally ran out when European veterinary experts failed on Monday to endorse an easing of the ban and allow exports of beef by-products such as semen, gelatin and tallow as recommended by the EU's executive commission.

5/22/96 BRUSSELS - "Major goes to war at last," screamed a front page headline in the Daily Mail, one of the newspapers portraying Britain as bravely standing alone and harking back to the darkest days of World War Two. Some European leaders could barely conceal their horror. Italian Foreign Minister Lamberto Dini spoke of "strong-arm tactics" and "blackmail". Swedish Foreign Minister Lena Hjelm-Wallen said it was not right to disrupt the work of the European Union, adding that she would not eat British beef.

5/27/96 LONDON - In a further setback to government insistence that British beef is safe to eat, independent health experts warned of a loophole in controls which could allow beef, that should have been destroyed, finding its way back into the food chain. The Chartered Institute of Environmental Health noted that farmers are able to take back the carcasses of cattle slaughtered in the government's mass cull program if they say the meat is to be eaten by their immediate family. But the health officers report said that meat could be sold on to the public by unscrupulous farmers prepared to break the law.

5/27/96 LONDON - Doctors and consumer groups accused the British government of a cover-up over evidence that leading brands of baby milk contains chemicals which could impair fertility. "Mothers will find this very frightening," said Dr. John Chisholm of the British Medical Association. They have a right to know the facts so that can choose milk that is safe." The Consumer's Association accused the government of putting commercial interests first. Fears about falling human fertility were first raised by a Danish scientist who in 1992 discovered that sperm counts among 15,000 men in 20 countries had dropped by almost half in 50 years.

5/28/96 LONDON - Anxious British parents deluged doctors and advice groups with calls for information Tuesday as a scare over formula baby milk posed another food safety crisis for a government already struggling with mad cow disease. The government and food manufacturers refused to name the nine brands of baby milk found in newly released test results to contain tiny traces of phthalates, a chemical which could impair fertility. The industry is investigating how the phthalates, which are used to soften plastics such as PVC, found their way into the powdered milk. The baby milk furor is the latest in a series of health scares which have panicked British consumers, including salmonella in chickens and eggs and listeria in soft cheese.

5/22/96 LONDON - British beef farmers and exporters today dismissed Prime Minister John Major's threat to paralyze European Union affairs over the mad cow disease crisis as "blood and thunder" that would not save their industry. While the government concentrated on trying to get the ban lifted, it had done little to help eradicate the disease or alleviate the financial impact on their industry.

5/25/96 LONDON - British electricity generating companies may be asked to help ease the backlog in the government's culling programs to eliminate mad cow disease. The Financial Times said the companies were carrying out urgent tests for the government to see whether they could burn rendered bonemeal and fat from cattle carcasses in power stations. It quoted Roger Freeman, minister in charge of the culling scheme, as saying in an interview that the government was seeking "radical options" for disposing of cattle remains, to start easing a 150,000 backlog of animals awaiting slaughter. "There is no way we can use conventional incinerators because that capacity isn't available," said Freeman.

5/30/96 GENEVA - The European Union complained today that some countries were barring British milk products, wrongly extending a worldwide ban by Brussels on exports of meat and meat products from Britain over "mad cow" disease. The sources said the official, whom they did not name, did not identify the countries which had moved against milk and milk products. A diplomat from an EU member state said there were several, but also did not name them.

5/31/96 ROME - Italy said it had developed an anti-mad cow disease test capable of detecting animal protein in feed destined for animal consumption. The ministry said that the test, which highlights the presence of any bone tissue components in animal feed by microscopic analysis, would ultimately be able to pinpoint what animal any of the proteins had come from.

6/3/96 BRUSSELS - Britain scored a partial victory in its fight against a worldwide ban on its beef products when EU farm ministers set the stage for the European Commission to lifting the ban on gelatin, tallow and bull semen. The farm ministers voted by nine to six in favor. It outlined British steps to reinforce measures to eradicate BSE, including making it a crime to possess feed which is blamed for the spread of BSE among British cattle.

Foreign Minister Klaus Kinkel said there was no way Germany could follow Brussels by easing or lifting the embargo, and Chancellor Helmet Kohl said public health took priority over the economic consequences of the ban.

The Berliner Morgenpost daily alluded to the anti-German rhetoric of British tabloid newspaper, commenting: "Suddenly it's the British, usually so proud of their pragmatism, who are hung up on principles as if they were the Teutonic ones." Referring to British Foreign Minister Malcolm Rifkind's insistence that Bonn obey EU law by following the commission's decision and ease the ban in Germany for certain beef derivatives, it added: "That's rich. London not only allowed mad cow disease to become an epidemic at all by playing it down for too long. It has now also got its way, not with superior arguments, but by blockading EU decision."

A commentator on national ZDF news said the easing of the ban showed that "blackmail pays." "Have experts produced new evidence? No. Has the number of mysterious deaths fallen? No," commented the mass-circulation Bild, under the headline "Politics Triumph Over Knowledge." "But the EU still decides to let British beef products be exported again, because the English applied massive pressure."

The Bonn daily General-Anzeiger accused the British of forgetting who was responsible for the crisis by portraying itself as the victim of Europe's injustice. "They just don't want to see that the embargo is not the result of malice but of concern for the welfare of consumers and farmers," it said, adding that Britain continued to take the view that "We are right, Europe still has a lot to learn." "This narrow-minded egoism evokes the arrogant rage of a driver on the wrong side of the motorway who fumes alone at all the traffic coming the other way," it said.

6/5/96 BRUSSELS, Belgium - The European Commission decided Wednesday to ease a ban on British beef exports but told Britain to end a controversial "beef war" on Europe if it wants all curbs ended. European Commission President Jacques Santer said shipments of gelatin, tallow and semen would only resume once the EU's executive was satisfied that Britain had fully complied with strict production rules and controls. Officials said this could take several weeks. Both sides still looked far apart in a bitter war of words, reflecting a crisis of confidence on beef, driven by health fears over mad cow disease. Britain, which says the herd disease is being eradicated, remained defiant toward its European Union partners, vowing to keep blocking EU business until a plan is agreed to lift a worldwide ban on its beef exports.

6/5/96 DIJON, France - German Chancellor Helmut Kohl said that public health had priority over any easing of the ban on British beef products over mad cow disease. The first and most important commandment must be public health before the economic consequences. A German official earlier quoted Foreign Minister Klaus Kinkel as saying there was no way Germany could ease or lift the embargo on British beef products for domestic political reasons. He quoted Kinkel as telling French Foreign Minister Herve de Charette that easing the ban was "not politically achievable" in Germany because of public and parliamentary health concerns.

British Foreign Minister Malcolm Rifkind issued a thinly-veiled warning to Germany not to unilaterally block the import of British beef and beef derivatives if the European Union eased its ban on the products. He said any national block on imports by Germany would violate European Union law.

6/5/96 LONDON - Calves could inherit so-called mad cow disease even if they were born after the feed ban intended to stamp out the notorious brain disorder, a team of British scientists warned today. Researchers at Oxford University said their study predicted that 75 percent of future cases of BSE will be found in animals born after the nationwide feed ban. They said signs of a shorter incubation period for BSE suggested maternal transmission, but they did not rule out calves contracting the disease through contaminated feed.

In an interview with BBC television's "Newsnight" Southwood who heads Oxford's zoology department, warned that hereditary BSE may be more widespread than previously thought. "If we know that calves from infected mothers are getting it, then they should be traced and culled so we can eradicate BSE from the British herd and restore public confidence." "I think public confidence in beef is not going to be fully restored, certainly not outside Britain, until we can show that we have very few cases occurring in our cattle herd," he added.

Britain's agriculture minister has failed to reassure his European counterparts that a limited slaughter of cattle over 30 months old would eradicate BSE. The Oxford study, if conclusive, could prompt calls for a wholesale cull.

6/6/96 BONN - German media today slammed Britain for failing to show more readiness to compromise after the European Commission eased a ban on British beef products, and said Bonn was right to maintain its tough stance. Health and environment conscious Germany is the leading skeptic on Britain's attempts to curb mad cow disease which, it is feared, may be transferable to humans.

6/6/96 PARIS - A French consumer association called for a boycott of British foods containing beef tallow or gelatin, following the European Commission's easing of an embargo on beef by-products from Britain. In the absence of a guarantee of the safety of beef by-products from Britain, UFC-Que Coisir calls on consumers to boycott all British food products containing tallow and gelatin . Que Coisir is a popular consumer magazine. The boycott would hit mainly biscuits, sweets and cakes, the consumer body said

6/7/96 PARIS - A leading scientist Dr. Dominique Dormont, a brain disease specialist, said in a report commissioned by the French government that mad cow disease is a potential threat to humans, echoing similar warnings in Britain. The report concludes that BSE should be assumed to carry an infection risk pending further research, which could take two years. "We have to give enormous importance to the possibility of human infection," Jean-Francois Girard, Director-General for Health at the Health ministry, told a news conference.

6/7/96 BONN - A quarter of German consumers have temporarily abandoned beef completely and up to 50 percent have reduced consumption in favor of other meats in the wake of 11-week old mad cow crisis, a survey showed today.

6\7\96 LISBON - British Foreign Secretary Malcolm Rifkind, winding up a six-nation European Union tours said he was hopeful a deal could be struck in the next two weeks to end the crisis over the mad cow disease. While the tone of the tour has been one of friendly persuasion, Rifkind had strong words for those EU countries which held out against any easing of the beef ban. He said that he was "deeply disappointed" by Portugal which joined Germany and four other countries in voting against an easing of the ban at a farm ministers' meeting last week. "There was no serious suggestion that it was because of any difference in scientific view," he said. "It seem to have been dictated by local political feeling," Rifkind said, adding that Britain wanted to take politics out of the issue and make it a purely medical and scientific matter.

6/8/96 PARIS - France's opposition Socialists, urging tougher measures to protect the public from mad cow disease, called for a continuing ban on imports of British beef products. Socialist Party spokesman Francois Hollande made the appeal after the European Commission voted earlier this week to lift a ban on British exports of beef gelatin, tallow and sperm but not the ban on beef itself. "The government, the authorities must take all the precautions necessary so that no products which might threaten the health of consumers enter the country" Hollande told reporters.

6/8/96 BRUSSELS - The European Commission said it had invited veterinary and public health officials from 68 countries to a Brussels seminar on Monday to discuss mad cow disease and measures taken to protect human and animal health.

6/8/96 BONN - One of Germany's most flamboyant politicians slammed anti-European Britons for having the gall to launch a hate campaign against Germany after covering up the health risks of British beef. "What bothers me . . .is that our friends the Britons covered up for years the fact that the meat they export to us is afflicted with pathogens that make you ill," Lower Saxony state premier Gerhard Schroeder told North German Radio. "This came to light and the European Union -- and that means above all Germany -- pays billions to limit the damage," added the Social Democrat whose unbridled political ambition and outspoken manner as often raised hackles in Germany. "And in the third step -- as gratitude, so to speak -- you see the worst hate campaign against Germans in the country since the war. I start to wonder who needs such Britons?"

6/9/96 CHEW MAGNA, England - Beef farmer Robert

Cowburn was so depressed by Britain's mad cow crisis that he killed himself. Just two days after returning from a market where prices had plummeted, he was found dead in his fume-filled car. Farmers are angry and confused. They say the government has done too little, too late. Germans are singled out as the bogeymen of Europe for their refusal to eat British beef. "If you start burning carcasses in a field, people will never eat beef again without tasting smoke," warned auctioneer John Wakeham. A party of Germans visiting the western English village of Wellington enraged the locals when they asked to be served chicken, turkey or fish -- anything as long as it was not beef. "The Germans are hypocrites. They are stirring it up but they have shot themselves in the foot. Their own beef sales have slumped," farmer Harold Carnell said.

6/9/96 LONDON - National Power is working on a feasibility study to test whether carcasses of cattle can be ground down into pellets and burned in power stations to generate electricity. The company said it was looking at substituting coal, which is usually used in its power stations, for pellets made from tallow and other cattle remains. The British government has been faced with a huge problem in disposing of cattle carcasses since it introduced a slaughter policy to combat mad cow disease. This has left the country with hundreds of thousands of cows that cannot be eaten. At present, carcasses are burned in incinerators but they have been overwhelmed by the number of cattle being culled, which has already exceeded 100,000.

6/9/96 BRUSSELS - The European Commission has drawn up a consumer guide on mad cow disease in which it pledges to keep the public fully informed about research. "The primary objective of the Commission is to safeguard public health and to keep consumers properly informed". It said the public was rightly worried because contaminated animal tissues -- the brain, spinal cord, retina and parts of the intestines -- have in the past entered the food chain.

6/9/96 BRUSSELS - Consumer confidence collapsed after

London said in late March that the deadly cattle brain disease, known as mad cow disease could be transmitted to humans. "The measures put in place to eliminate contaminated cattle feedstuffs were highly unsatisfactory, allowing contaminated feed to be used even after regulations were introduced," the European Trade Union Confederation said.

6/9/96 LONDON - European Commission President Jacques Santer has warned Britain the rest of Europe is turning against it because of its policy of refusing to cooperate with its partners in protest at the export ban on British beef. In a bitter attack in an interview published in Sunday's Observer newspaper, Santer also accused British ministers of "absurd" behavior which would leave the country isolated for years. "We are coming to the hour of truth, and going as far as the limit of our possible tolerance. It is not just governments, it is public opinion, consumer organizations, pressure groups and lobbyists. I have to say that the British government has been responsible for mismanagement of the whole crisis."

6/10/96 LONDON - British farmers could face jail if they fail to get rid of banned cattle feed believed to be a cause of mad cow disease, the government announced. Farmers are being told to surrender feed made with the remains of sheep and cattle and the government is offering $9 million to finance the recall operation.

6/11/96 BERLIN - German Health Minister Horst Seehofer said that Germany would consider taking legal proceedings against the European Commission after it agreed last week to lift a ban on exports of some British beef bull semen, gelatin and tallow. "All sixteen states joined in opposing the decision of the EU. We will make our decision (over whether to sue) within the next two months," Seehofer told the news conference. He said he was still convinced that British beef products could pose a risk to public health.

6/11/96 LONDON - Restaurants from Singapore to Vienna are assuring anxious diners that British beef is off the menu as worldwide fears of mad cow disease show no sign of abating. Despite a ban on exports of British beef, the biggest food scare to hit the country in years has reached around the globe and caused devastation at home. Health-conscious Germans are horrified at the thought of even the slightest risk that they might catch Creutzfeldt-Jakob disease, the fatal human equivalent of Mad Cow disease. Beef consumption has fallen by a third, despite reassurances from Britain that its beef is safe. Germans are now eating more pork, game, poultry, fish and even horse meat -- almost anything, in fact, as long as it is not beef. A party of Germans visiting the west of England farming town of Wellington had to be smuggled secretly into the homes of local families with whom they were staying. The Germans from Bavaria requested that they be fed no beef during their stay and organizers feared ugly scenes if they arrived openly. Many Britons themselves have reacted to the ban by deciding it is their patriotic duty to eat beef.

6/11/96 BRUSSELS - Britain and its partners are in an angry dilemma over their "beef war," pressured on all sides, and without the luxury of much time to sort it out. London says firmly it will not stop disrupting EU business until it gets a step-by-step plan for lifting the worldwide ban on its beef. The rest of the EU, furious at what it sees as "absurd" behavior by Britain and still unconvinced by Britain's BSE eradication plan, is increasingly reluctant to submit to what it sees as "blackmail." Posing an even greater difficulty, continental consumers, frightened of eating British or any other beef, are pressuring their governments not to relent. One of the two sides will have to blink to avoid the bitter split many fear is coming in Florence.

6/11/96 PARIS - Mad cow disease gripped the French parliament on Tuesday when Agriculture Minister Philippe Vasseur traded accusations with the Socialist opposition of putting public health at risk. Riled by heckling from the opposition, Vasseur accused the Socialists of having allowed beef from herds where cases of bovine spongiform encephalopathy (BSE) had been found to be sold in France when they were in government before 1993. "You put meat from those herds on the market. So shut up!," Vasseur bellowed at the Socialists. "If you climb up a tree, you should make sure your pants are clean," he said, citing a saying from his northern home region. Nation Assembly speaker Philippe Seguin had to call repeatedly for order during an acrimonious question time. "Since the beginning of this crisis, our concern at every moment has been to preserve public health," Vasseur said. "In the next few days...we will offer a bill to the assembly on the safety and hygiene of food products." The agriculture minister also accused the Socialists of having allowed animal feed containing bonemeal, a suspected cause of BSE, to be fed to French cows.

6/12/96 TEL AVIV - The science journal Nature reported on Wednesday that Britain more than doubled exports of potentially contaminated animal feed after banning use of such feed itself. Israel imported nearly 10,000 tons of British feed in 1991 and Thailand 6,200 tons, the journal said. But according to Arnon Shimshoni, director of veterinary services at Israel's Agriculture Ministry, in 1991 Israel bought British feed made only from chickens.

6/12/96 BRUSSELS - Britain renewed efforts to defuse the "beef war" with its European Union partners on Wednesday, offering a new plan for the gradual ending of a worldwide ban on British beef. Senior EU veterinary officials, however, underlined difficulties in solving the crisis by demanding that Britain slaughter thousands more cattle than it had planned. London has infuriated its partners by initiating a policy of disrupting EU business until it gets what it wants.

Key British demands, such as allowing sales of calves born after May 1, 1996, and cattle from grass-fed BSE-free herds, would remain in the blueprint which sets out steps for progressively ending the ban. British officials, meanwhile, said they were dismayed by the vets' demand that more animals be slaughtered. "We have been against including the 1988/89 year because it is going to be very difficult to do. It goes back before animal birth certificates were introduced," a British diplomat said. It extends a program started in May to slaughter and burn one million cattle over 30 months old that may have eaten contaminated feed.

6/12/96 LONDON - Citing government statistics, Nature said tens of thousands of tons of feed that could have included the remains of infected animals were exported after a 1988 ban on using it in Britain. The British agriculture ministry confirmed the report, but said anyone who bought feed containing the ground-up remains of animals knew its use was restricted in Britain and knew why.

British government scientists believe that Bovine Spongiform Encephalopathy (BSE or mad cow disease) is caused by feeding cattle the remains of sheep infected with scrapie, their own version of the deadly, brain-wasting disease. They banned the use of such feed in 1988, and have tightened restrictions on what can be fed to animals since then. "They knew at the time that meat and bone meal was dangerous, yet they exported it and spread the danger of new cases of BSE arising in member states," Udo Weimer, a German agriculture ministry official, told the journal.

But a spokesman for the Ministry of Agriculture, Fisheries and Food said no subterfuge was involved. "We were exporting feed up until 1990 which would have contained parts of cattle," the spokesman told Reuters. "The European commission knew what we were doing at the time, and the other countries knew. They didn't feel it was a problem...They knew that we were not feeding that stuff to cattle and sheep and it was up to them what they fed it to." He said the feed was considered safe to be fed to pigs and chickens, although Britain has banned its use completely and will make it illegal to produce or use animal feed containing bone and meat meal from mammals. "There is a lot of lying around and we announced on Monday we would be collecting it and destroying it," he added.

Francis Anthony, a spokesman for the British Veterinary Association, said his organization questioned the export of feed that was forbidden in Britain. "I remember posing the question was it moral to export feed which was perceived to be a poisoned feed?" Anthony told Reuters. "I was told that everyone knew about this and it was the "buyer beware syndrome." Anthony pointed out that while there had been 160,000 cases of BSE in Britain, there had only been about 400 in other countries. "If we accept the food-borne theory of BSE, there should have been many, many more cases. We are now six years down the line and we would have expected a fair number of cases by this time," he said. "We've either got cases being concealed or we've got cases incubating and about to show up or it's not food-borne. And one thing we are pretty sure of is that it's food-borne." Since BSE was first identified in 1986, many people have been horrified to learn that natural herbivores like cows have been fed sheep, other cows and even bits of bone to boost their meat and milk production. Although the practice is more than a century old, some farmers say they did not know what was in the feed. Mark Savay, a professor of pathology at the Center National d'Etudes Veterinaires et Alimentaires near Paris, said other countries snapped up the British feed because it was cheap. Prices plummeted once the British ban took effect.

Britain said it will provide an extra four million pounds ($6.1 million) for research into mad cow disease which has infect its cattle and resulted in a worldwide ban of its beef by the European Union.

6/13/96 BRUSSELS - The European Commission, which is trying to broker a deal to avoid an angry and divisive summit on June 21 and 22, firmly put responsibility for controlling the use of British exports of meat and bonemeal animal feed on member states.

"If member states did not control the use to which meat and bonemeal feed was put then that was their responsibility," Commission agriculture spokesman Gerard Kiely said.

A spokesman for Britain's Ministry of Agriculture, Fisheries and Food said no subterfuge was involved in the exports. "We were exporting feed up until 1990 which would have contained parts of cattle," the spokesman told Reuters. "The (European) commission knew what we were doing at the time, and the other countries knew. They didn't feel it was a problem...They knew that we were not feeding that stuff to cattle and sheep and it was up to them what they fed it to." He said the feed was considered safe to be fed to pigs and chickens, although Britain has banned its use completely and will make it illegal to produce or use animal feed containing bone and meat meal from mammals.

6/13/96 PARIS - Scientists warned the European Commission in early March of the risk that humans could be contaminated by mad cow disease but were pressured into silence, the French newspaper Le Monde reported on Thursday. Le Monde published extracts from a March 8 report by the commission's Food Science Committee, stating: "The risk of human contamination by tissue infected with BSE still exists." It quoted an expert on the committee, speaking on condition of anonymity, as saying; "At our March 8 meeting, we were subjected to very strong pressure from General Directorate," (the commission department in charge of agriculture). "They wanted very clearly to prevent us from delivering that opinion. We were told such an opinion would worry the population unnecessarily. But we stood firm. It was very tense and we parted in anger," the unidentified expert said. Asked what had happened to the document, he said: "It was put on the commission table and we never heard of it again." Le Monde said the same committee had subsequently warned the commission on April 15 of the risks of easing the embargo by allowing the sale of three British beef derivatives -- gelatin, tallow, and bull sperm. It took that decision last week.

Outrage swept France Thursday after the disclosure that Britain authorized massive exports of animal feed suspected of causing mad cow disease, much of it to France, after banning its use at home in 1988. The influential daily Le Monde called the British feed sales an "industrial crime." Commentator Pierre Georges said, "It's people who are really mad, not just cattle. Mad for profit, mad for unbridled market liberalism."

He said the British mentality was "Sell, sell at any price." "The Crime of the English", the popular daily France-Soir concurred in a banner headline. "The English stuffed us with their feed," it screamed. Wednesday Britain confirmed a report in the scientific journal <u>Nature</u> that said it exported tens of thousands of tons of feed that may have included the remains of infected animals after a 1988 ban on using it domestically.

The leader of France's most powerful farm union, Luc Guyau of the FNSEA, said he was outraged by the disclosures and vowed to do everything to ensure the British beef ban stayed in place. He told Reuters Television that anyone involved in importing suspect feed should be tracked down and brought to court if fraud had been committed.

French government scientists said Thursday they had found the first experimental evidence of a link between mad cow disease and its human equivalent, Creutzfeldt-Jakob disease (CJD), in work on monkeys. Two neurologists working for the Atomic Energy Commission and the French army health service said their research showed striking similarities between brain lesions in monkeys injected with the crushed brains of cows infected with bovine spongiform encephalopathy (BSE), and a new form of CJD observed in humans. Their study, to be published by the British scientific <u>Nature</u>, lends new weight to the theory that BSE can be passed to humans, although they stressed it did not prove that.

Scientists Corinnne Lasmezas and Jean-Philippe Deslys said they had injected the brain concentrate into two adult macaque monkeys and a newly-born one in 1991. Three years later, all three began to show behavioral disorders -- anxiety, nervousness, and depression -- and had developed identical brain lesions and died. The scientists, who had been studying BSE, said they had only been alerted to the possible link with CJD by the British announcement and had the compared their results with new cases of the human disease observed in Edinburgh, Scotland, in mid-May.

Deslys said the brain lesions were "very close, strikingly

similar" and constituted "a first experimental argument for a casual link between the bovine illness and the new form of CJD in the British patients." He said the lesions were flower-shaped patches surrounded by cavities. The researchers said they injected the concentrate directly into the monkeys' brains rather than giving it to them orally. They declined to say firmly whether BSE can be transmitted to humans but said their findings called for further research.

6/13/96 LONDON- Dutch veterinary doctors said on Wednesday they had developed a test which might lead to the early detection of mad cow disease and its human equivalent. BSE and CJD can now be diagnosed for certain only after the victim dies. The brain is dissected and checked for the typical sponge-like holes.

Veterinary doctor Bram Schreuder and colleagues at the Institute for Animal Science and Health at Lelystad, Netherlands, said their test could help officials trying to control the spread of BSE. They noted that animals with spongiform encephalopathies all had an altered brain protein known as a prion. They also knew that antibodies to these prions showed up in lymph tissue in scrapie-infected sheep as early as 10 months of age, years before they appeared in the brain.

"We have now detected mutated prions in the tonsils of sheep in the preclinical stage of the disease, long before the onset of clinical signs," they wrote in the science journal Nature.

6/14/96 BRUSSELS - Possession of feed containing meat and bone meal will be made a criminal offense from August 1.

6/14/96 PARIS - Leading British retailer Marks & Spencer, in a move certain to raise eyebrows in London, ran ads in major French newspapers Friday to assure consumers it sold no British beef or beef products in its French stores.

The advertising campaign followed last week's easing by the European Commission of an export embargo of British beef, imposed in March over fears of mad cow disease, to allow sales of tallow, gelatin and bulls' sperm in the European

Union.

Marks & Spencer, seen in France as an icon of all that is typically British in taste, booked quarter-page advertisements saying in bold capitals: "No derivatives of British beef are used in our products." "No article currently sold in Marks & Spencer's French shops contains derivative products of British beef, notably beef gelatin of British origin," said the retailer, whose food halls are wildly popular in France.

Customs statistics published on Friday showed that after France banned British bonemeal from being fed to cattle in 1989, purchases dried up. But import resumed in 1993, ostensibly to be fed to pigs and chickens, and continued until March 1996.

6/16/96 BONN - British animal feed potentially contaminated with the agent that causes mad cow disease was still being delivered to Germany years after Bonn had imposed a ban on its import, according to the news magazine Der Spiegel. In a report released ahead of publication, Spiegel said official British export statistics showed 22.7 tons of feed containing animal remains was exported to Germany last year alone, in defiance of a 1989 ban.

6\16\96 PARIS - French media have reported that beef sales have gone down by over 25 percent since the mad cow crisis began. "I have seen people on the verge of suicide, who have lost practically all they had," said Agriculture Minister Philippe Vasseur . Asked what would happen if France lifted its ban on British beef, he replied: "If tomorrow we lifted the embargo against Britain . . . the French wouldn't buy any meat at all."

6/16/96 VIENNA - The Austrian government on Sunday called on Britain to end its blockade of European Union business imposed in protest against a ban on British beef, warning the move endangered European integration. The EU embargo was eased last week when the European Commission allowed exports of gelatin, tallow and semen to resume. Austria was among several EU members to vote against a partial lifting of the ban at the end of last month.

6/18/96 PARIS - France banned the sale of sheep meat infected with the disease scrapie on Tuesday in a widening public health crackdown triggered by the mad cow crisis, the agriculture ministry said.

The French national meat council said farmers were obliged to declare cases of the disease and the new measures could lead to the slaughter of entire flocks of sheep where a single case was reported, a policy already in force to combat BSE in cows.

The disease has not previously been considered a danger to humans, but there is mounting scientific evidence that infected sheep may transmit it to cows. A science ministry official said Vasseur's ban was a precautionary measure, already in force in Switzerland. "I can promise you one thing: protecting French citizen's health will be Jacques Chirac's sole concern in Florence and if we have to show solidarity with a member state, it wouldn't be at the price of endangering French citizens and consumers."

6/18/96 BONN - Germany may seem the toughest of all European Union states when it comes to protecting its citizens against any health risks posed by BSE "mad cow" disease. But in the country itself, many people think the government is not informing them adequately or fighting hard enough in Europe's "beef war" to keep the fatal cattle disease at bay.

"Since the BSE scandal, many consumers want to know exactly what sort of meat they are eating and precisely how BSE can be transmitted," said Beate Dussa, who runs a BSE telephone hotline -- one of many set up recently across the country. Dussa is being bombarded with questions" Can you catch BSE by eating fruit or vegetables cultivated using cattle dung? Can you catch BSE through gelatin used in the manufacture of medicines, food products or cosmetics? Is it safe to eat poultry which could have been given feed containing BSE-infected cattle remains? Can mad cow disease be transmitted through bull sperm? "It's frustrating for us all, because the an-

132

swer in most cases is 'We just don't know'," said Dussa. "There is no scientific proof either way. That's why consumers are changing their habits and turning more to ecologically-farmed meat."

One survey found a quarter of consumers have temporarily given up beef, while nearly half have reduced beef consumption in favor of other meats. And even when the rest of the EU made a concession to Britain by lifting the ban on some beef products, the German regional states were firm that as far as they were concerned the ban on British beef was still in place. The Bonn government is considering taking its case against re-admitting the products to the European Court of Justice.

6/18/96 BRUSSELS - The European Commission will oppose an early resumption of British beef exports to non-EU countries in a revised framework plan aimed at a gradual lifting of the worldwide ban, EU sources said on Tuesday. "Exports to third countries will be permitted in parallel to phased exports to other EU member states." But the EU source added that in view of continued strong public health fears of Germany, Austria and other member states, a resumption of British beef exports to EU member states, and therefore non-EU countries, was unlikely for some time.

The European Court of Justice is due to hear on Wednesday Britain's request for an interim ruling to suspend the worldwide ban. Some member states were also concerned about the moral question of dumping British beef, considered unfit for EU consumers, on poor countries. Resumption of beef exports to African, Asian and other non-EU member states was one of the main points of the original five-stage framework plan presented by Britain to the Commission on June 11 for a phased lifting of the ban. The other stages are a resumption of exports of cattle embryos, calves born after September 1, 1996, beef from grass-fed herds certified to be free of mad cow disease and of meat from animals under 30 months old. Britain would first have to remove all meat and bone meal from animal feed.

6/19/96 LONDON- The agent that causes mad cow disease may still be getting into cattle feed because of sloppy procedures by animal food producers, a BBC television program said on Wednesday. It said the discovery could explain why British cattle are still becoming infected with mad cow disease, seven years after cattle feeds containing animal remains were banned. The Newsnight program quoted a 1994 agriculture ministry report saying that 42,000 tons of deadly offal, potentially infected with the mad cow agent, could not be accounted for. One gram (0.035 ounce) is enough to cause bovine spongiform encephalopathy -- mad cow disease or BSE. Newsnight said such feeds were banned in 1989, but 60 percent of all cases of BSE-- 27,000-- were in cows born after the ban.

It said that inspectors from the Ministry of Agriculture, Fisheries and Food had found breaches of regulations designed to prevent BSE contamination were widespread at all levels of the feeds producing industry. Farmers believed the missing offal had been used in feeds for pigs and poultry and the infection had passed into cattle feed somewhere along the production line. This may have taken place at the abattoir, renderers or in the food mill, Newsnight said.

National Farmer's Union official Anthony Gibson told the BBC: "If it hadn't been in pig and poultry feed it wouldn't have spread into cattle through cross-contamination. We would not have had the 25,000 cases born after the ban and we wouldn't be in the dreadful state that we are in with Europe."

6/19/96 OSAKA, Japan - A Japanese interior goods sales company said Wednesday it has voluntarily recalled British soap made from cow oil although the company did not find the soap was related to "mad cow disease." The company just finished recalling some 1,700 bars of soap from retailers nationwide, leaving the company holding 7,900 bars. It sold 23,000 bars before it stopped selling the soap.

Japanese government officials banned products containing British beef in April after reports of a suspected link between mad cow disease and a human brain disorder surface in Britain earlier this year. Japan imported 199 tons of bladders and stomachs, 17 tons of other internal cattle organs and 106 tons of pet food containing beef from Great Britain in 1995.

6/19/96 BRUSSELS - The European Union headed on toward ending the "beef war" as Britain gave way to a key EU demand -- killing more cattle at risk from mad cow disease-- before lifting a global ban on British beef. Commission President Jacques Santer said: "It's an ethical problem" when referring to the fact that it would be unfair to sell British beef to people in poorer countries outside the EU when it was judged unfit for European consumers. Britain says it is not attempting to dump its beef on poor countries but to sell food that is eaten by millions of Britons to countries that want to buy it. The Commission's framework for a step by step removal of the ban included only exports of meat from grass-fed BSE-free herds, cattle embryos, animals born after a specified date, meat from animals under 30 months and in the longer term meat from animals over 30 months of age.

6/20/96 PARIS - France plans to compensate farmers forced to destroy sheep infected with scrapie, a malady similar to mad cow disease, the Agriculture Ministry said on Thursday. The ministry disclosed on Tuesday that it had added the degenerative nerve illness in sheep to a list of contagious diseases subject to strict veterinary controls. The step meant French farmers must report all cases, and meat from infected sheep must be kept out of the food chain. The Lyon- based National Veterinary and Nutritional Center (CNEVA), which is already conducting research on BSE, will also study scrapie, ministry sources said. The 200-year-old disease had not been previously considered a danger to humans but there is mounting scientific evidence that infected sheep may transmit it to cows.

6/20/96 LONDON- John Collinge, and expert in BSE-type diseases at ST. Mary's Hospital in London, said there was another problem in predicting any epidemic. "We don't know what foods it (the infective agent) went into," he said. "We know that one gram of brain can kill a cow. We need to know how many grams people are exposed to in a typical British diet." Some scientist say tens of thousands of people could have been infected with BSE and predict an epidemic of CJD, which has a long incubation period, over the next 30 years.

6/21/96 FLORENCE - At a summit meeting in a red-brick Florentine fortress, the 15 EU leaders reached a compromise reconciling Britain's demand for an end to a worldwide ban on its beef exports with other EU states' insistence on strict public health guarantees. In response to Britain's demand to be allowed to export to third countries beef that was banned from sale to EU partners, it was agreed the European Commission would examine such request case-by-case on the basis of scientific advice.

6/21/96 PARIS - French farmers clashed with police on Friday in a day of protests to demand European Union aid for beef producers hit by falling sales in the mad cow crisis.

Five policemen and three farmers were injured in the northwestern city of Le Mans. There were more clashes in Tulle, capital of President Jacques Chirac's home Correeze region, and at the Channel port of Ouistreham where farmers tried to stop a British ferry from docking.

French beef sales have fallen by up to 30 percent since March when Britain said there may be a link between bovine spongiform encephalopathy (BSE) --mad cow disease-- and its deadly human equivalent Creutzfeldt-Jakob Disease.

The protests coincided with an EU summit in Florence, Italy, where heads of government agreed a deal to end the British beef export ban and London's blockade of EU business.

Police and farmers went into a war of words after trading tear-gas grenades and petrol bombs in Le Mans. FNSEA blamed the police for aggressive tactics in firing tear-gas grenades which seriously wounded three farmers. The national police union called the protesters irresponsible.

In other protests, farmers burned an effigy of British Prime Minister John Major outside the European Parliament in the eastern city of Strasbourg late on Thursday. They threw eggs and firecrackers at police in the northern town of Rouen.

6/21/96 BONN - German Foreign Minister Klaus Kinkel said on Friday Bonn's demands had been met by an EU summit deal allowing a phased lifting of a ban on British beef while opposition Social Democrats attacked the agreement.

Agriculture Minister Jochen Borchert held out little hope that all restrictions on British beef exports would be lifted soon... adding that, for this to happen, Britain must prove that its cattle were no longer being fed with contaminated animal meal, and that all cows likely to have been infected had been slaughtered with no risk of further infection.

6/25/96 LUXEMBOURG - Around 1,200 angry farmers from across Europe besieged a meeting of European Union farm ministers Tuesday noisily demanding full and immediate compensation for losses caused by the mad cow crisis.

Farmers from Italy, France, Germany, Belgium, Luxembourg, Ireland and Britain exploded fire crackers, burned tires, sounded sirens and hosted a wreath to their "departed revenue" above the entrance of the ministerial building.

Luc Guyau, President of the French national farmer's union, shouting to make himself heard above the wailing sirens and exploding fireworks, warned that more aid would be needed in three months if the crisis was still raging. The EU must take urgent measures to restore the beef market, consumer confidence, and exports to countries outside the EU, he said. "It's a question of aid but above all of confidence."

6/26/96 LONDON - In a letter to the science journal, Nature a study showing monkeys can develop a new strain of the human version of mad cow disease after being injected with brains from infected cattle was published.

Corinne Lasmezas, a neuro-virologist at the Atomic Energy Commission, and the colleagues at the French army health service said they had injected brain material from BSE- infected cattle into the brains of two adult macaques and one newborn. Nearly three years after inoculation "the two adults developed abnormal behavioral signs including depression for the one, edginess and voracious appetite of the other." They also started to show the difficulty in moving and tremors that typify the disease.

The baby monkey showed signs even sooner. All three were killed and their brains examined. They had deposits of the abnormal prion protein, a mutated brain protein that most scientists think causes the diseases. The pattern was "strikingly" similar to that seen in the new CJD cases but different from the pattern seen in the brains of macaques that had been infected with normal CJD from humans. Although the monkeys were injected the researchers said there was probably no difference between having the infectious agent injected and eating it. Other tests have shown the abnormal prions survive very high temperatures and would likely make it through the digestive system unscathed. Adriano Aguzzi, a neropathologist at University Hospital of Zurich, said it was worrying that the small amounts of cow brain material used in the experiment infected the monkeys.

"It is unsettling that these amounts are well within range of brain tissue  present in commercial food products for human consumption until a few years ago," he wrote in a commentary in Nature. "On the other hand, however spectacular (and worrying) these findings are...we can hope that the oral route of administration will be considerably less efficient.'

6/26/96 LONDON  - Britain said on Wednesday it would start publishing numbers of cases of the human form of mad cow disease four times a year, instead of annually, because of the huge interest in the disease. Sir Kenneth Calman, Britain's Chief Medical Officer said "Clearly, with the present intense interest in the disease, there is a need to put statistics into the public domain more frequently."

7/4/96 PARIS - A Paris court threw out charges by Belgian meat producers that French beef labels meant to reassure consumers over the British mad cow crisis were a protectionist ploy that damaged Belgian exports. The court dismissed the case, targeting Agriculture Minister Philippe Vasseur, saying the ministry had only given "logistical support" for an initiative by French meat producers. And it said consumers had the right to know the origin of their food.

7/5/96 LONDON - French researchers said they had discovered what they believe to be the first case of a non-laboratory monkey catching a form of mad cow disease. The researchers, writing in the Lancet medical journal, said the discovery appears to back up theories that mad cow disease can be transmitted between species through the food chain. The monkey had been fed on meat products. The only monkeys previously reported to have contracted BSE were deliberately infected in laboratory experiments. This monkey was fed on standard monkey food, including one containing meat products declared fit for human consumption. The monkey developed the first symptoms of spongiform encephalopathy, lethargy and mood swings. The research team from the University of Montepellier wrote that as far as they are aware, this is the first reported case of spontaneously developed spongiform encephalopathy in a monkey.

7/8/96 DUBAI - Six Gulf Arab states have decided to keep their ban on imports of British beef and beef products as part of measures to combat the spread of mad cow disease, United Arab Emirates (UAE) newspapers reported on Monday. They said this was agreed at a recent meeting of Gulf Cooperation Council (GCC) members Saudi Arabia, Bahrain, Kuwait, Oman, Qatar and UAE in Riyadh.

7/8/96 BRUSSELS - European Union Farm Commissioner Franz Fischler said on Monday he was checking reports that British beef was being sold illegally to Italy and other continental countries. The press reports said German Health Minister Horst Seehoffer had called for an EU inquiry after being tipped off by the German ambassador in Rome about large scale cheating on the EU's export ban imposed in late March.

7/8/96 PARIS - A herd of 75 milk cows was recently destroyed in the Mayenne department of western France after the discovery of a case of mad cow disease in the herd, the agriculture ministry said on Monday. "The case was the eighth in France this year and the 21st since 1990," a ministry spokeswoman said. Virtually all the cases discovered in France have been in the west of the country, especially in Brittany.

7/10/96 BONN - The German cabinet agreed to extend indefinitely an emergency import ban on British cattle, beef and beef products imposed in March because of fears of mad cow disease, the agriculture ministry said. The Commission said shipments of gelatin and tallow would have to wait until it was satisfied that Britain had conformed with strict production controls.

7/12/96 ROME - Italy urged its European Union partners to step up vigilance in their beef controls after reports that British beef was being smuggled in via other countries in defiance of an EU export ban. According to some reports, British cattle due to have been slaughtered were loaded in Scottish ports and shipped to Italy.

7/12/96 PARIS - France has banned its farmers from feeding any protein extracts from animals but will particularly affect the use of fishmeal and poultrymeal in fodder given to cows and sheep. "The use of meatmeal, bonemeal or both, and any protein of animal origin except for milk products, is forbidden in the feeding and manufacture of ruminants whatever their age," the text of the decree in France's Official Journal said. Paris had already banned animal feed producers from putting bonemeal made from bovine carcasses into cattle fodder. But until now, farmers have been able to feed it to pigs, poultry and fish -- some of which themselves end up in cattle feed as part of the industrial feed chain. French authorities had previously insisted there was no scientific evidence that pigs, poultry or farmed fish would widen the risk of mad cow disease by eating tainted feed and then passing it back to cattle. Industry figures show that between 5,000 and 10,000 tons of fishmeal, and 30,000 tons of poultrymeal, are fed to cows or sheep in France each year.

7/13/96 BRUSSELS - The European Court of Justice rejected a second British bid to lift a European Union global ban on Britain's beef exports, cause of international jitters over mad cow disease. The president of the Luxembourg-based European Union Court of First Instance, Antonio Saggio, acting on behalf of the full court said the European Commission had not over reached its jurisdiction in imposing the ban and that, on the contrary, it had a responsibility to protect public health. On the issue of the ban on exports to non-EU countries, Saggio said there was a significant danger that British beef could be re-exported into the EU.

7/16/96 PARIS - France on Tuesday launched a plan to tighten rules on the use of beef derivatives in lipsticks and other cosmetics to shield against fears of transmitting mad cow disease to humans. "One can't say (cosmetics) are completely risk-free because they can be applied onto wounded skin or together with products that favor transport through the skin," Secretary of State for Health and Social Security Herve Gaymard said. He told a news conference that he would take steps in coming days to force cosmetics makers to use only beef products from herds free of the disease, to exclude cow organs most associated with the disease and to tighten factory processing rules. Cosmetics firms use numerous beef derivatives, including fats, spinal cord and placentas.

7/19/96 LONDON - A London court ruled today that the British government had been negligent in the cases of some children who developed the human equivalent of mad cow disease after being treated with the human growth hormone As the medical warnings increased in 1977 the health department decided that because there had been no cases of CJD (human equivalent of mad cow disease) the judge told the court the "risk of contamination was too awful to contemplate or at least should not be the subject of public knowledge or discussion."

7/19/96 BONN - Germany's upper house voted today to

extend an import ban on British beef, beef products and cattle because of fears about mad cow disease which could put Bonn on a collision course with the European Commission. The upper chamber representing Germany's 16 regional states amended a government bill regulating British beef imports to forbid the import of bull semen-- one of three by-products on which the commission has lifted an import ban. The commission has ruled that the substance is safe and said that any country refusing to allow it to be imported would be breaking European law.

7/22/96 TOKYO - Dainippon Pharmaceutical Company said Monday it was recalling three imported drugs for the treatment of anemia and bronchitis due to the possibility that they contain fat extracted from cattle in Britain. The Company said it had began collecting 400,000 pills of Fero Gradument, a drug for the treatment of anemia, and 140,000 cylinders of Medihaler Iso and Medihaler D, for bronchitis. The drugs are manufactured by Abbott Laboratories Ltd. and 3M Health Care Ltd. and imported by Dainippon.

7/22/96 BRUSSELS - A new health scare broke in Europe's crisis over mad cow disease when scientists warned that the brain-wasting condition could spread directly to sheep. European Union Farm Commissioner Franz Fischler disclosed that research indicated that what looked like the centuries-old sheep disease scrapie could actually be BSE (mad cow disease). He said that by introducing the agent which causes the disease in cattle to sheep, scientists had found it could spread more widely in sheep that in cattle. The disease had infected both spleens and nervous tissue in sheep, whereas in cows only the nervous system was affected.

8/2/96 PARIS - The French scientist credited with isolating the virus that causes AIDS says humanity could face an onslaught of killer diseases on a scale even larger than the current epidemic, which has infected 14 million people. CJD, the brain wasting human equivalent of mad cow disease, was just one of the new breed of ailments that had the potential to do massive damage, he said. "The recent examples of AIDS and mad cow disease should remind us we're living in a dangerous world," Montagnier said. CJD was a huge potential threat. "The potential worst scenario is that you could have thousands of people lying sick and dying of this disease," he said.

8/4/96 LONDON - A British government spokesman denied on Sunday that fresh tests had been ordered into the safety of milk after a newspaper reported fears that it could become infected with mad cow disease. The observer newspaper said government scientists were conducting urgent tests to ascertain whether cow's milk could be infected with Mad Cow disease. Earlier tests were unreliable, it said.

8/5/96 BONN - German Agriculture Minister Jochen Borchert said the German government and all states have all agreed that the European Union's scientific committees must swiftly assess whether there are any possible risks in milk," he said. Baerbel Hoehn, environment minister of North Rhine-Westphalia -- Germany's most populous state -- suggested that British milk products might have to be banned in light of findings that cattle could pass the disease to calves. She told German radio, the European Union had already erred by relaxing its ban on British beef products and should now consider restoring or even tightening the restrictions. "We should seriously consider if we should not restore the stricter import ban that used to apply, or whether we should not extend it to milk products," said Hoehn, a member of the Greens party that is in opposition in Bonn.

8\6\96 BONN - Health-conscious Germans wary of the dangers of mad cow disease turned a worried eye to a new source of alarm -- British milk and cheese. Consumer watchdogs and some state officials demanded British dairy products be banned in light of a new study suggesting cows might pass the disease to calves, raising the nightmare scenario that milk could carry bovine spongiform encephalopathy. George Abel, managing director of the Bonn-based Consumers' Initiative lobby group, said, "there should be an and European Union wide export ban on British milk and milk products," he told German Radio. "If this cannot be implemented in Brussels -- and there are good reasons to assume this -- then Germany must do it alone if necessary." Baerbel Hoehn, environment minister in Germany's most populous state of North Rhine-Wesphalia said. "I like to eat cheese and lots of it, but at the moment I would not eat any British milk products," she told Southwest Radio, reiterating her call for a British milk ban. She made clear there was still no proof that milk could carry the disease. "Nevertheless, as long as we cannot rule out this risk, I continue to believe it is better to be safe than sorry."

8/8/96 ATLANTA - U.S. health officials warned doctors today to step up their efforts to look for the human version of mad cow disease. Health officials will now investigate any deaths from CJD among people under age 55. "If you see something like this, don't just automatically assume that it's not CJD," said Dr. Larry Schoenberger a medical epidemiologist in the CDC's National Center for infectious Diseases.

SUMMARY

I hope these news reports have given you an insight of how politics works in agriculture. How different countries are more health conscious than we are. I commend Oprah Winfrey and the news media for airing much of this on TV and in the newspapers. I commend France for banning feeding ruminants, fishmeal and poultrymeal to cows. Let us do what we can to influence our government to do what is right.

# CHAPTER FOUR
# COW LEUKEMIA AND CANCER

Beware of the cow was the topic of an editorial over two decades ago in the Lancet of July 6, 1974. This prestigious British medical journal reported that infant chimpanzees fed unpasteurized milk from birth developed leukemia and pneumocystis carinii pneumonia. Twelve chimpanzees were removed from their mother at birth, nursed separately, and fed either unpasteurized Bovine leukemia virus, containing milk or a prepared infant formula (sterilized SMA). Only two of these chimps, Bois and Roger, received milk from the cow #BF044 whose milk had an abundant and constant source of Bovine leukemia virus (BLV). The most shocking aspect of the deaths of these chimpanzees is the disease state that they displayed at death. Erythroleukemia and Pneumocystis carinii pneumonia were diagnosed when they died at 34 and 45 weeks of age after a 5 to 6 week illness. These animals died of pneumocystis carinii pneumonia. This condition is the hallmark of AIDS. Bois and Roger developed leukemia drinking milk from cow #BF044. They also developed an immuno-deficiency that allowed the pneumocystis carinii pneumonia to develop. The chimps had white blood counts of 53,000 and 64,000. [76 77 78 79] In a word, the Chimpanzees had AIDS![80] The experimenters explained: "It seems likely that the Pneumocystis Carinii Pneumonia was secondary to the cancer disease, as is often the case in man.., probably resulting from immunologial deficiency incident related to the malignant disorder.[81] In one group of AIDS patients studied, 63% died after developing Pneumocystis carinii pneumonia. The chimpanzees susceptibility to infection with BLV is obviously additional evidence of potential human health hazards associated with BLV. [82]At autopsy both animals showed infiltration of neoplastic cells in the bone marrow, spleen, lymph nodes, lungs, liver and kidneys. Pathologists at both Emory University and the University of Pennsylvania, including Dr. Peter C. Noel and Dr. David T. Rowlands, Jr., a total of 11 pathologist concurred in the diagnosis. [83] When this experiment was performed it was before the HIV was discovered, and before AIDS. It is possible that cow #BF044 not only was infected with the Bovine leukemia virus but also the Bovine immunodeficiency virus (BIV or cow aids virus) before the virus was known or discovered in cows. This is probably the reason the Chimpanzees also developed AIDS. For confirmation the experiment should be conducted again with milk from a cow with both Bovine leukemia virus and the Bovine immunodeficiency virus and fed to baby Chimpanzees.

In one experiment nine lambs were injected with cell-free BLV, and all nine died of lymphosarcoma within 6.5 years. Virtually all cattle infected with BLV remain carriers for life. In another experiment newborn sheep inoculated with lymphocytes from cattle infected with bovine leukemia virus became persistently infected with BLV. Fifty percent or more of the sheep died with lymphosarcomas (cancer) confirmed by microscopic examination of cells. This provides definite evidence that BLV is a tumor inducing virus and demonstrates conclusively that BLV is a leukemia producing virus.[84] Experimental animals that die of BLV on autopsy have infiltration's of cancer in the bone marrow, spleen, lymph nodes, lungs, liver, heart, stomach, spinal cord, kidneys,and behind the eyes. [85] [86] In another controlled study, 5 of 42 sheep died after inoculation with BLV with microscopic confirmed lymphosarcoma (cancer).[87] a recent experiment in Sweden, calves infected with the bovine leukemia virus surprisingly showed no antibodies to BLV using the Polymerase Chain Reaction test (PCR). The PCR test provides a revolutionary tool, for the first time, to put the laboratory scientist in the drivers seat in an epidemic investigation. This is a novel discovery and can detect retroviruses RNA segments in milk. BLV proviral DNA was frequently demonstrated in the uterus, liver, kidney, stomach, and lymph nodes by the polymerase chain reaction (PCR) test.

The BLV proviral DNA was also found in urine, saliva specimens, and spleen . Amazingly these were detected by the Polymerase Chain Reaction test in animals infected but without circulating antibodies in their blood. This is of primary interest because humans can also have animal retrovirus present in their cells and even in cancer cells of tumors without having antibodies. [88] We can now better evaluate why antibodies were not found in humans 15 years ago. Polymerase Chain Reaction (PCR) is one of the most widely used molecular tools today because it enables the detection of retroviruses of Bovine leukemia virus infection at very low levels in milk, animals and cancers..[89]

Before going to medical school, I inspected dairies in Marin and Sonoma Counties in Northern California. I also was in charge of inspecting the Petaluma Co-op plant whose brand name was Clover milk. The Petaluma Co-op plant furnished milk to the City of San Francisco. During that time I enforced sanitation on dairy farms. I encouraged wells to be constructed properly and protected from contamination, and I also had many dairy farms install septic tanks for the farm houses. Strangely, the cows loved to drink the effluent from the sewage from the dairy farm houses. During my medical school years, 1962-1963, I worked as a milk inspector for Orange County, a large populous county just south of Los Angeles, and San Bernardino County, which is one of the largest counties in the United States. While in medical school I spent a large amount of time searching the literature regarding cows and leukemia in the Veterinary journals, I learned about the Bittner milk factor that revealed virus particles in the milk that was transferable to the baby mice from their mothers and caused leukemia. This stimulated me to search more in the literature, as I recalled the large lymph nodes I would see on cows during my inspection of dairy farms. The material on the infant chimpanzees developing cancer was reported shortly after my graduation from medical school. My oldest son, who had just been admitted to medical school tragically developed

Hodgkin's disease (a cancer disease of lymph glands). This combination of events motivated deeper interest in my research.

## INTERVIEW WITH DR. KELLEY DONHAM

In 1981, an interview with Dr. Donham,[90] a veterinarian with the University of Iowa, by the Journal of Health and Healing, touched on the question of the relationship between cancer of cattle and human leukemia. Dr. Donham stated, "We gave the BLV to eight chimpanzees and all eight animals turned up with antibodies to bovine lymphosarcoma in their blood. This kind of response indicated infection with the disease itself, not just reaction to vaccination. The only thing left to prove, beyond any shadow of a doubt, that the cattle disease was indeed transmitted to the monkeys, is to find the virus in the monkeys. So far, we have not been able to re-isolate that virus from those animals." To the question asked: Well, don't viruses have a well-known tendency to hide out for many years and be undetectable by any means, and then show up later? Donham replied: "That's right." "Dr. Donham, how do you suspect the cattle lymphosarcoma is transmitted from cattle to man? Milk? Meat?" Dr. Donham stated: "One possibility is milk. One of my graduate students here just finished a Ph.D. research about the ability of that virus to survive in milk. It does survive quite nicely. It is very highly associated with cells, and can survive within lymphocytes (one kind of white blood cell) in milk up to 3 days. We studied this under the conditions that milk is handled on the farm. Animals are usually milked by mechanical milkers and the milk goes straight to a pipeline into a bulk tank. It's cooled and it stays there for anywhere from one to three days until a milk truck comes, and picks it up and takes it to a processing plant where it is processed. Under those conditions of time and temperature storage, the virus does seem to survive quite nicely and remains infectious for that period of time. The majority of our milk today is pasteurized. But most dairy farm families just go out to that bulk tank and pour out what they need for the family and drink it unpasteurized. That's very common. In fact, in the survey we find between 70% and 80% of the farm families who have dairy farms do that. Another thing is that because of the increase of "organic influence" in food, a lot of people prefer unpasteurized (raw) milk because they think it is more wholesome. We know that probably in the neighborhood of about 13 million pounds of milk is consumed unpasteurized in this state of Iowa." The next question asked was: "There is certain to be lymphocytes in meat. Do you suppose that if meat is not thoroughly cooked, people could get this cancer from meat as well as milk?" Dr. Donham answered: "I think that's certainly a consideration. There was an article published in Lancet[91] several years ago that looked at different countries and meat consumption, and showed that the more meat the people of any country consumed, the more leukemia there was in that country. Whether the meat caused the leukemia has yet to be studied."

## PREVALENCE OF BOVINE LEUKEMIA VIRUS IN 1981

On October 1985 I presented a paper at the American Academy of Family Practice in Anaheim, California, included was much of the following.. Over a decade ago in the United States 20% or more of the adult dairy cattle and approximately 60% of dairy and beef herds surveyed are infected with BLV. Now it is thought that even 60% of the cows are infected with BLV due to the increase of cows coming to slaughter with Bovine lymphosarcoma. The incidence varied considerably from herd to herd, but herds having 80% or more infected adult animals are not uncommon. [92] Most BLV infected cows release infectious virus or infected lymphocytes in their milk.[93 94 95 96 97 98 99 100] Many cows culled from herds for poor production and other reasons have been found to have incipient or evidence of leukemia. [101]

## INCREASE OF LYMPHOMA IN CATTLE

I flew to Atlanta, Georgia and presented a poster on April

4, 1986 at the Preventive Medicine Conference for all the public health officers of the United States, which was well received. I then presented an hour lecture on raw milk and leukemia for the Western Milk and Food Conference at the University of California at Davis, attended by 400 of the top managers of the dairy industry. I received excellent comments from the dairy inspectors and members of the dairy industry who attended this lecture. Leland H. Lockhart, Chief, Milk and Dairy Foods Control of the California State Department of Food and Agriculture wrote me a letter saying, "on behalf of the Western Food Industry Conference, I wish to thank you for the excellent presentation you made on Raw Milk Consumption and Bovine Lymphosarcoma. This is a new subject to the dairy industry in California but is one which people who consume raw milk should be aware of."

BLV infection rate has reached up to 50% in those areas of Japan and Venezuela where Human Lymphotrophic Virus I(HTLV I), the virus causing Human T Cell Leukemia, is also endemic or uncontrolled in the human population. . Individual herds in these regions may have rates approaching 100%.[102] In Japan the complete sequence (the genetic makeup) of BLV has been reported and indicates an intimate relationship with HTLV-1 and HTLV-2, which infect humans. Because of the high prevalence of BLV infection in cows and the high prevalence of leukemia in humans in Japan it causes further suspicion that BLV could cause cancer and leukemia in humans.

## EPIDEMIC OF CANCER IN CALIFORNIA

In California annual culling for slaughter due to various reasons is estimated at 25 percent of adult dairy cows.[103] It was reported in 1985 that an epidemic of lymphosarcoma in dairy cows is occurring in California and in the United States it is increasing at an unprecedented rate. Mature cows slaughtered in 1990 for Bovine lymphosarcoma caused by BLV was, triple the level found in 1975.[104] [105] Moreover, rates of condemnation for Bovine lymphosarcoma may have been underestimated here to the extent that moribund or sick cattle were not acceptable for slaughter and were not examined after death, and were rendered and fed back to cows and other animals. In 1981 more than 47%-almost one-half-of 7,768 dairy cattle in Florida were found to be infected with BLV. This was the highest concentration of BLV in the world except Venezuela.[106]

Of 100 cows infected with the BLV approximately 30% will develop persistence Lymphocytosis. This is a rise of the absolute lymphocyte (a kind of white blood cell) count in the cow and it will remain elevated for approximately 4-5 years where upon 30% of the cows develop Bovine lymphosarcoma (cancer). During the time of persistent lymphocytosis there is a shedding of live BLV in the milk with a resulting in an increase of number of somatic cells (pus) in the milk. In any case there probably is an increase of the lymphocyte count in the milk and because of the increase somatic cell count in the milk many of these cows that have mastitis may actually have BLV infection.

## STATEMENT OF THE PROBLEM

BLV is frequently present in raw milk and lymphocytes containing the BLV genome and can be absorbed directly in the intestines into the blood stream. Proviral DNA may be present in hard unpasteurized cheeses and not inactivated by the aging process, and also present in pasteurized milk as shown by the Elisa test and the Polymerase Chain Reaction test.

BLV is shed in the milk so that many people are drinking, milk that contains a virus that can infect or cause cancer in other animals including the Chimpanzee, pig, sheep, and goat and possibly others. This virus has been shown to infect human cells in the laboratory.

There is no reason to doubt that BLV prevalence is continuing to increase. It remains to be seen how high the rate of infection must rise before, the threshold for industry action, is reached for an eradication program. We have been talking about it for over a decade.

We must have milk from cows without cancer and BLV. This is the opinion of many in the medical profession. Dr. J. F. Ferrer, along with others, is concerned about the proviral DNA that has inserted its RNA into the lymphocytes and that it may survive pasteurization in a transformed lymphocyte. Studies comparing the tumor characteristics of lymphoma in humans and lymphosarcoma in cows show that they are similar. Another reason to eradicate infected cows is that people who live around large herds of cows with BLV may become infected with BLV by biting flies.

## CHILDREN DYING OF LEUKEMIA

It has been noted that, compared with many other neoplasms, there is a relatively high incidence of fatality of leukemia in children, with two small but persistent peaks in children aged about 3 and adolescents aged about 17. It appears that exposure to infection may play a greater part in the generation of this disease (leukemia) than has yet been demonstrated.[107] [108] [109] [110] [111] [112] As we all know nearly all children drink milk and the main food in infancy is milk. The plausibility that BLV may be a risk factor in leukemia in children and Hodgkin's disease and Lymphomas in young adults is extremely high. From birth to death the probability of developing Invasive cancers is 1 in 2 in males, and in females it is 1 in 3.[113] Breast Cancer Action, an organization of breast cancer survivors and their supporters, reports that 182,000 women were diagnosed with breast cancer in 1993. That there were 46,000 deaths from breast cancer in 1993, which translates into one death every 12 minutes. The incidence has more than doubled in the past thirty years. One in eight American women will be diagnosed with breast cancer during her lifetime. And no one knows why.

Why are more and more women getting breast cancer in the first place? I feel that it is related to epidemic of Bovine leukemia virus in cows and the presence of the BLV even being produced in the breast of the cow. It would be so simple to have a compulsory eradication for the Bovine leukemia virus like that in so many European countries. This is a Public Health problem that can be reduced by using preventive medicine. Approximately 70% of the dairy cows get meat-and-bone meal from cows in their diet. The primary problem is that there is no feed labeling, so the farmers do not know what they are feeding. The public should insist that these despicable practices stop. How important each of these women was to dozens of people--family, friends, coworkers, students, clients, neighbors--now left stranded by her death.

## GETTING THE PROBLEM TO THE PUBLIC

I practiced Family Medicine in Bakersfield, California for 3 years and then moved to Ashland, Oregon in 1971. I continued to evaluate studies and literature involving BLV in cows and became more interested in the study of the Epidemiology of Cancer. In 1981 I began postgraduate studies in Cancer Epidemiology. I was granted a Public Health traineeship to work on my Doctor of Public Health at the School of Public Health, Loma Linda University. All of my work was funded by this traineeship. Dr. Howard Ferguson agreed to oversee my practice in Medford, Oregon while I was in Loma Linda. At first I tried seeing patients on Mondays and Fridays, and getting up at 4:00 a.m., driving to Sacramento, and taking a flight to Ontario, California, arriving at 10:00 a.m. for classes. I stayed in my son's room Tuesday and Wednesday nights at the men's dormitory. This became more difficult and after 6 weeks we obtained a U-haul trailer and moved down to a condominium at Loma Linda. After the first year I presented a lecture at the Alumni convention of the School of Public Health on the Bovine leukemia virus. This was before the HIV (AIDS) virus was discovered. Dr. Marjorie Baldwin heard my lecture and asked me to write an article for the Health and Healing journal. The cover displayed a Holstein cow with the word "cancer" written across its lateral side. After this talk I was asked to speak at many other meetings. I attended a meeting in San Diego in which Dr. Robert Gallo, head of the Laboratory of Tumor Cell Biology at the National Cancer Institute of the National Institutes of Health, reported on his research on the AIDS virus. After the meeting I had a long conversation with him regarding the Bovine leukemia virus. He encouraged me to send him blood samples from patients with a strong history of consuming raw milk and that had come down with leukemia.

### CROSSING THE SPECIES BARRIER

It is noteworthy that leukemia proved contagious not only from cat to cat, and from monkey to monkey, but also from cow to monkey. This crossing of the species barrier is alarming since the milk of a viremic cow fed to newborn chimpanzees was capable of transmitting the disease in a very short time. Although extrapolation to man is difficult, the distances are getting dangerously shorter. The presence of some bits and pieces of viral RNA genes causing comparable diseases in mice and primates has been implied in 48%-91% of human leukemia's, 69%-75% of human lymphomas and sarcomas, and 30%-67% of human breast cancers. Simultaneous detection of reverse transcriptase and a high molecular weight RNA in human malignancies is further evident for the causal presence of RNA viruses in human tumors.[114]

Many doctors and health professionals believe we will see a reduction in all types of cancer in humans, especially those cancers in humans related to fat consumption, when we wipe out BLV in cattle. We should take the present evidence available and eradicate BLV which is simple and economical to do. A test to detect BLV in milk used in Europe can be applied to bulk tank milk or individual animals.

There are large numbers of leukocytes, macrophages, lymphocytes and other blood cells prevalent in milk. Milk codes encourage not over 750,000 cells per cubic centimeter (5 cubic centimeters =1 teaspoon) of normal milk. It is possible that humans who may resist small amounts of lymphocytes infected

154

with BLV virus may have their immunity overcome by inoculation with very large numbers of live lymphocytes. For example, animals die after an injection of 100 live tumor cells, while immunized animals may survive injections of 100,000 or even 1,000,000 live cells. But they will still die from cancer if 10,000,000 live cells are injected. When immune responsiveness is reduced, control over environmental antigenic stimulation is less effective and a chronic antigenic bombardment of the lymphoid system results. This continued uncontrolled irritation of the lymphoid system causes malignant changes resulting in increased frequency of lymphoid cancer. Immunosuppressive treatment may also activate otherwise latent endogenous viruses (viruses sleeping in the body), and lymphoid cancers occur as a result of immunosuppression. [115]

Since it is possible that the human immune system may be overcome by large amounts of lymphocytes present in milk and by ingesting large amounts of milk. The amount of consumption of milk and dairy products by the individual may be the deciding factor whether BLV causes cancer in humans. There may be a significant difference between an individual who drinks two glasses of milk per day and one who drinks one to two quarts of milk a day. The same may be true of the individual who consumes one pound of cheddar cheese per week as compared to an individual who consumes one pound of cheddar cheese per month. Rare beef may not have reached a temperature high enough to inactivate the infectivity of BLV. And we know that Epidemiology studies have shown that eating beef gives an increased risk of colon cancer

Pasqualini brings out the difficulty of making a prognosis in lymphoproliferative processes (like leukemia, Hodgkin's, and multiple myeloma). Patients with the same cancer cells in the blood often follow a very different course, some die in a very short time while others survive for many years and a few are even cured. One is often under the impression that there must be a (still to be discovered) triggering factor involved. On the one hand, the pathogenic effects for man of certain zoonosis have been little explored, not only in relation to intimate contact with sick animals, but also to the ingestion of infected animal foods, including chicken and fish. On the other hand, viral, bacterial or parasitological infections, may play an important part in the etiology of neoplastic transformation (of cells turning cancerous).[116]

## PASTEURIZATION AND BOVINE LEUKEMIA VIRUS

An article in Science in 1981 by Dr. J. F. Ferrer from the Microbiology Department of the University of Pennsylvania really inspired me to keep working. He brought out the following information. There is no evidence that BLV can infect humans, but neither does the data exclude this possibility. Although attempts to demonstrate BLV antibodies, particles, and antigens in humans have been negative, the findings are not conclusive because of the limited sensitivity of the assays used and because some BLV-infected cells do not synthesize virus particles or viral antigens.[117] [118] [119]

Pasteurization seems to destroy the infectivity of BLV in milk, but the effect of pasteurization on the nucleic acid of BLV is unknown. Moreover, it is not known whether pasteurization destroys the biological activity of the proviral BLV DNA in the infected cells in milk.[120] Bovine leukemia virus must survive the approximate one-half hour transit time through the acidic medium of the stomach and gain access to the surrounding tissues. Recent research has shown that lymphocytes from milk gain access to the tissues by passing through the intestinal wall. Study using radioactive labeled lymphocytes in nursing rats and their eventual appearance in peripheral blood supports this contention.[121]

Milk is defined as a lacteal secretion, practically free from colostrum, obtained from the complete milkings of one or more healthy cows. Cows infected with a large number of retroviruses, such as BLV, and with cancer are not healthy cows. Pasteurization, even though greatly responsible for the reduction of food-borne disease outbreaks from milk, has not eliminated possible public health problems in this area.[122]

## VIRUSES SURVIVE PASTEURIZATION

I attended a conference in Keystone Colorado for one week where the top Epidemiology students from the nation were gathered for a week to be taught by the top pathologists and scientists in the nation on the etiology of cancer. There I met Dr. R. J. Rubino who had just completed his doctoral thesis on BLV under Dr. K. J. Donham at the University of Iowa. We discussed BLV at length and he sent me his thesis which had not yet been published .

While working on my Doctor of Public Health degree in Cancer Epidemiology I was also an Associate Professor of Family Practice at the School of Medicine, Loma Linda University and there I taught Junior Medical Students. I instructed the medical students as much as I could about the Bovine leukemia virus even though I knew that they would not be asked questions on BLV on the National Boards. This was also new material to the doctors and teachers at the School of Medicine and the School of Public Health. In the microbiology department, Dr. Robert Nutter, a virologist, encouraged me in my work and was a great help in reviewing my research.

Investigations have shown that milk can be a protective medium for certain viruses, for example, foot and mouth disease virus, maloney leukemia virus, rauscher leukemia virus, rous sarcoma virus and the bovine papilloma virus survive pasteurization.[123] Our present pasteurization temperatures are archaic and should be upgraded to kill as many viruses as possible. DNA viruses survive heat better than RNA viruses.

The exposure of the US population to unpasteurized cheese (e.g., Swiss or blue cheese) is widespread and risky, as these cheeses may contain BLV, or proviral DNA of the BLV, after the aging process of cheese. [124] Present technology cannot produce any raw milk or raw aged cheese that can be free of human pathogens.[125] Nearly all tumors, leukemia's, and lymphomas in many cold-blooded and warm-blooded animal species thus far investigated have been found to be caused by transmissible viruses. Rather than speculate on a different etiology of the same disease in humans, it would appear more reasonable to assume that human tumors, lymphomas, and leukemia's are also caused by transmissible viruses.[126]

Most Swiss cheese is not pasteurized; ice cream may be a product that BLV might appear to survive as BLV appears to survive at colder temperatures. The higher solids, (excluding fat, whey, and dry milk products) in a milk product will require a higher temperature to kill or denature viruses. Remember pasteurization is not a cover up for unsanitary milk. Only 99.9% of bacteria are killed during the process of pasteurization. Certain bacteria can survive both extreme cold and heat.

## DENIAL

The dairy industry becomes extremely defensive when the effectiveness of its pasteurization methods is questioned. It is interesting to note that the tobacco industry has for years denied any relation of lung cancer to cigarette smoking. Today the dairy industry completely denies that the bovine leukemia virus can be of any harm to humans.

## BLV PRODUCED IN THE UDDER OF THE COW

Even before the discovery of BLV there were virus-like particles that had been identified by electron microscopy in the milk. Now there is startling evidence that BLV is present in the mammary organ of the cow more commonly called the udder of the cow. BLV is actually present in the glandular cells that produce milk in the udder of the cow. In infected cows these antigens are expressed in the udder of the cow while the cow is being milked. It has been proven beyond doubt that this production occurred in mammary epithelial cells. The investigators cited that their most effective tool was their PCR data using primers from the unique pX portion of the BLV genome (the part that the virus uses to start cancer in a cell). This region is not found in any other retrovirus except human T cell leukemia viruses, which, like BLV, are exogenous viruses. Exogenous retroviruses are not inherited genes passed from your infected ancestors. BLV has traditionally been thought to be present only in the lymphocytes of infected cows as a silent infection. Now the evidence shows that BLV is also present in the mammary (which is the breast of the cow) epithelial cells and expresses antigen in vivo (living animal) in this cell type. These antigens could also stimulate antibody production, and might account for the fact that dairy cows more frequently have detectable BLV antibodies than beef cattle. [127] The discovery that the glandular cells in the cow where milk is produced actually have cancerous viruses where the milk is produced is astounding. This nearly unimaginable cause can only serve to intensify our fears concerning the transaction of cancer between cows and humans.

## BOVINE LEUKEMIA VIRUS INFECTIONS

Bovine leukemia virus infections in cows are associated with decreased dairy production and a shorter life span. For practical reasons in both the United States and Europe, these cows are usually sent to slaughter and removed from that herd before any clinically detectable signs of the disease emerge.[128] The Bovine leukemia virus establishes a persistent infection in lymphocytes (a type of cells in blood) of cows by inserting bits of genes of proviral DNA at a number of sites in the lymphocytes DNA. The majority of infected cattle remain healthy for life, although approximately 30% develop a lymphocytosis (huge numbers of lymphocytes in the blood, like leukemia in humans). A proportion of these, about 10% develop Lymphosarcoma , (cancer that affects every organ of the body.)[129] Of BLV infected cows with persistent lymphocytosis 25-35% of the total lymphocytes harbor BLV viral genes. It is my opinion that when you drink milk that contains these lymphocytes you are setting yourself at risk for leukemia, lymphoma, Hodgkin's disease, multiple myeloma and multiple sclerosis or other cancers related to fat such as prostate, breast, and colon cancer, even if the milk is pasteurized.

## BOVINE PAPILLOMA VIRUS

The bovine papilloma virus has been isolated from commercially available milk at retail outlets and is not inactivated at present pasteurization temperatures. Two milk samples from six separate dairies revealed particles indistinguishable from bovine papilloma virus and no significant reduction was obtained during pasteurization for two hours. This indicates that bovine papilloma virus transformation capabilities occur at temperatures in excess of pasteurization of milk. In essence, this virus survives all currently practiced levels of pasteurization. Experimentally, bovine papilloma virus (BPV) will induce tumors in the bovine brain and urinary bladder and BPV will also produce sarcoid-like tumors in horses. The Syrian hamster developed fibromas and fibrosarcomas of the skin, chondromas of the ear, meningiomas in the brain, after inoculation injection of BPV. Metastasis to the lung occurs in approximately 10% of BPV-induced hamster tumors.[130] In humans, one kind of papilloma virus is thought to be responsible for cancer of the cervix in woman.

## INTERRELATIONSHIP OF BOVINE LEUKEMIA VIRUS WITH OTHER VIRUSES

It has been shown that the human AIDS virus and BLV can be activated by other viruses such as the herpesviruses, and that other factors may also activate retroviruses, such as continual antigenic stimulation.[131] It can be speculated that when milk contains many different viruses they could activate the cancer process in humans. Aids can be transmitted by blood in humans. Cows have Bovine AIDS. Milk contains blood and blood cells. The Human AIDS Virus, The Cow AIDS virus, and the Bovine leukemia virus are all retroviruses and have similar properties.

Proliferating cell nuclear antigen (PCNA) has been shown

to be associated with human leukemia and malignancies. Patients with leukemia, chronic myeloid leukemia, carcinoma of the breast, colon, lung, kidney, stomach, skin, ovaries and testes, and neuroblastoma tumors all had high levels of PCNA in their cancer cells. When sheep were infected with lymphocytes containing Bovine leukemia virus the PCNA was significantly increased in sheep lymphocytes as a result of BLV infection. This provides evidence that PCNA has a role in the development of cancer in sheep as result of BLV infection.[132] Since PCNA is also elevated in many cancer cells of humans, could it be because humans have ingested PCNA in milk containing BLV lymphocytes?

Unfortunately, catastrophes do occur in which pasteurized milk is accidentally contaminated with raw milk. One of the worst related dairy disasters hit the Chicago area in April of 1985. 180,000 illnesses were linked to the outbreak. This is another reason to eradicate the Bovine AIDS virus and the Bovine leukemia virus in milk. This pasteurized milk which people drank would also have been contaminated with BIV and BLV.[133] Although milk is pasteurized it may still be contaminated with raw milk due to human mistakes in the pasteurization of milk. Eradicating BLV and BIV would indeed be preventive medicine and excellent public health policy in the highest sense of the word because it would enable us to have milk from healthier cows.

## CANCER SECOND LEADING CAUSE OF DEATH IN CHILDREN

Malignant diseases are the second leading cause of death in the United States in children, with leukemia accounting for about 50% of all childhood cancer deaths. Certainly, all milk served to our children and adults should be free of leukemia virus, and produced from leukemia-free cows. Legislation requiring pasteurization of milk and cheese and a compulsory eradication program of bovine leukemia virus in dairy cattle is needed. BLV is a disease amenable to complete eradication, as has been done in other countries

## LETTERS AND PROGRESS

While carrying on my active Family Practice in Medford, Oregon, I spent an entire summer writing to every U.S. Senator and Representative in Congress regarding BLV. Dana, my daughter in-law, had recently moved from Fargo, North Dakota with my grand children, Laura and Amy, after Don, my son had died at the age of thirty-six. He had had a heart attack in 1986 from the radiation he had received to his chest 8 years before to treat his Hodgkin's disease. This waste of a brilliant young doctor further impressed upon me that something had to be done to stop cancer from robbing us of our best young people. I started on an intensive letter writing campaign to scientists in the country to inform then of BLV. I searched the literature at many universities like University of California at Davis, California Polytechnic College at San Luis Obispo and Pomona. I received some favorable letters from Senators who referred my letter to the USDA and FDA. I feel that some good accrued because it did educate some of the legislators. However, the dairy lobby is so strong that because of politics and the lobbyists donating money to certain Senators and Representatives not much could be accomplished. One improvement was made with the prohibition by the FDA of the interstate shipment of raw milk.

## CONFOUNDING EVIDENCE

Although not proven, there is an ample reason to speculate that it is the retroviruses from animal sources rather than the fat itself that is the reason for many human cancers such as breast, colon, prostate, lymphomas and leukemia. Why do I say this? Epidemiologists use the term confounding. Let me illustrate. If I should do a study on lung cancer, I could randomly examine 100 people's second and third fingers. Those fingers that were stained yellow I would find these persons to have a twenty times greater chance of developing lung cancer than those with no stains on their fingers. We know that it is not the yellow stains on their fingers that caused these people to develop lung cancer, but the fact that the yellow fingers came from holding cigarettes while smoking. It was actually the cigarette smoke that was the culprit in lung cancer. It may be that confounding is deceiving us into believing that it is the fat that is causing certain kinds of cancer when it really is the retroviruses that are causing cancer. Epidemiology studies done in China, in certain areas where the populations do not have meat or dairy products, show that they also have very little cancer, osteoporosis, or heart disease.

Cancer costs Americans 15.3 billion annually according to Dr. Robert W. Hoffman of Washington State Blue Shield. Non-medical costs for caring for children with cancer are already so high that some families are forced into bankruptcy. Thomas A. Hodgson, Chief economist for the National Center for Health Statistic said 1.25 million Americans were diagnosed in 1980 as having cancer. He said that the total cost for cancer_care was 15.3 billion dollars. I say if we eradicate Bovine leukemia virus and Bovine Aids virus we would reduce the incidence of cancer. We would have fewer Medicare bills and this would go far in the fight to balance the national budget and reduce the national debt.

## HUMAN LEUKEMIA CLUSTER CASES

Occasional clusters of leukemia have shown various unusual epidemiological features which are difficult to attribute to chance. Miles, a suburb located just North of Chicago, between 1957 and 1960, experienced eight cases of childhood leukemia representing a 15-20-fold increase over the expected incidence. Seven of the eight cases occurred in Roman Catholic families. Each of the families concerned had one or more children attending the community's one parochial school and they drank the milk supplied to them at school. The eight cases occurred in two distinct time periods. A similar time period was observed among eight cases of apparent acute rheumatic fever which occurred during the same four years among children attending the parochial school. These cases rep-

163

resented four times the incidence of rheumatic fever seen in the public school children from the same neighborhood. The appearance of rheumatic illness also suggests a relationship in this community between leukemia in children and some infectious process.[134]

Another leukemia case came to the attention of the CDC in 1968 when a 16 year old son of a dairy owner died of lymphosarcoma progressing to acute lymphocytic leukemia. Ten years earlier a hired hand of this farm had died of lymphosarcoma progressing to chronic lymphocytic leukemia. A case of chronic lymphocytic leukemia was found in a neighbor whose property adjoined the farm and leased his land to the dairy farm for grazing stock. Several months after the investigation began the diagnosis of chronic lymphocytic leukemia was made in a second neighbor whose property also adjoined the farm. The dairy herd in question consists of approximately 250 Holstein cows. Lymphosarcoma has occurred for many years in this herd at a frequency of perhaps one case per year.[135]

Between 1970 and 1973, seven cases of acute lymphocytic leukemia were diagnosed in Elmwood, Wisconsin. This represented a 20-fold increase in expected incidence. A number of patients had either worked or lived near the town creamery. The manufacturing milk powder and processing whey occasionally pervades the air of the town and even frosts the nearby trees.[136]

Cancer has been diagnosed in eight members of a farm family in Connecticut in contact with BLV infected dairy herd. Diagnosis included two cases of ovarian cancer, two of uterine cancer, and one each of leukemia, Hodgkin's disease, lymphoma, and stomach cancer. [137]

A few cases of leukemia have been reported in farmers whose cattle had lymphosarcoma. In one instance, a farmer had "lymphadenosis" for 7 years. Two years after his disease was apparent, 25 of his cows had lymphocytosis and 6 months later, 7 cows died with lymphosarcoma. In Germany, a son of a farmer whose cows had Bovine leukemia, had drunk raw milk for years. He developed leukemia and died at the age of 30. In the same report, the author mentioned that leukemia developed in another owner of a small Bovine leukemia-affected herd. Lymphatic leukemia was reported in a father and son who worked in a creamery and had contact with a farm where there was Bovine leukemia in the cattle. Other observations were of leukemia patients from farms and a case of Hodgkin's disease in a person who lived on a farm where bovine leukemia was diagnosed 2 years later. It has also been observed that rural residents of California had a slightly higher risk for leukemia and Hodgkin disease than did urban residents.

I attended a 6 week course in Minneapolis on Epidemiology. There, Dr. Alfred S. Evans from Yale University and author of Viral Infections of Humans was a classmate of mine when we received our Masters of Public Health degree at the University of Michigan in 1959. He took me aside and said I should consider going to Japan to study the HTLV I Leukemia in humans and BLV which is endemic in Japan. I was not able to do that as I had to keep my practice going in Medford, Oregon. Dr. C.W. Heath was one of the instructors there and he reviewed an article I had written on the Bovine leukemia virus and gave me suggestions. We also discussed cluster cases of leukemia he had investigated while at CDC. I believe he later went to the American Cancer Society.

## LEUKEMIA IN DAIRY WORKERS

About 1981 a Twin Cities television station for Minneapolis and St. Paul, Minnesota on its late news telecast presented a four part series on the bovine leukemia virus and its possible human health implications. The series was developed in response to a question presented by a Minnesota dairy farmer whose young son had developed leukemia. In attempts to determine the source of his son's illness, the father became concerned that the raw milk the family consumed might have been responsible. In addition, the dairy farmer studied the county records in which he found that over a period of several years that other young children had died from leukemia and they also had a history of consuming raw milk. The four part series attempted to inform the viewing audience about bovine leukemia and its possible public health importance. In response to this the Extension Veterinarian put out a news letter to County Extension Directors with the following information. It reported that the human lymphoid leukemia mortality rates for the rural states of Iowa, Nebraska, South Dakota, Minnesota and Wisconsin are statistically significantly higher than the US average. Exposure to cattle has been suggested as a contributing factor to human leukemia. He also stated that over 2000 human sera have now been examined for antibodies to BLV and that they had all been negative. From this it was concluded that there is no epidemiological or serological evidence from human studies to indicate BLV can infect man. [138] Because of these studies an eradication program for BLV was never enacted and the American public was never warned of the dangers of Bovine Leukemia being transmitted by milk. We now know, however that the assumptions from these studies were limited because retroviruses have now been found to have infected humans.

## A FATAL MISTAKE IN JUDGMENT

Caldwell [139] reported in one seroepidemiologic study of farm families and their dairy herds, 145 persons were in contact with and drinking unpasteurized milk from 30 BLV-infected herds(as measured by antibodies to BLV) and 47 people were reported in 6 persons in contact with a seropositive herd; the difference was not statistically significant. None of the 192 people had antibodies to BLV. Using the gel diffusion test for the internal p23 BLV antigen. Antibodies were not found in 80 Wisconsin veterinarians with extensive contact with cattle, in 15 workers in a laboratory, in 5 farmers with BLV-infected dairy herds, and in about 100 human patients with various forms of leukemia. In another study, 73 Iowa veterinarians and 30 people with leukemia also were negative by gel diffusion test, using p24 antigens. The same study also included investigation of 21 dairy herds in which lymphosarcoma occurred, and 33% of the cows were positive for BLV, but there were no positive reactions to BLV antigen in 45 people on these dairy farms even though 35 of them consumed raw milk.[140] Another study using the complement-fixation test for BLV antibodies, negative results were obtained in 400 human serums from matched controls and cancer patients, including 93 with adenocarcinoma, 51 with squamous cell carcinoma, 9 with undifferentiated carcinoma, 11 with melanoma, 7 with small cell carcinoma, 14 with Hodgkin's disease, 3 with lymphosarcoma, and 14 with sarcoma.[141] [142]

The foregoing studies revealed no BLV antibodies found in humans so CDC (Center for Disease Control) decided it was not a public health problem. All of the public health programs were based on this study. Bovine leukemia was allowed to disseminate to epidemic proportions in our cows. Unfortunately, now all the foregoing conclusions to the outmoded tests are to no effect since we have Polymerase Chain Reaction test (PCR). We need to now repeat these studies using the more accurate PCR test on human serum or blood, and can also detect the proviral DNA of retroviruses in humans. We can now make new public health policies and decrease the incidence of cancer in our population. The future will be determined by you the consumer, what action you will take, what you eat, what letters you write. Do not underestimate your power and your influence.

## DEATHS IN AGRICULTURE WORKERS

Causes of death among 1,551 white male veterinarians were compared with the general United States population. Among veterinarians in clinical practice, the proportion of deaths was significantly high for particular neoplasm's (cancer) especially leukemia and Hodgkin's disease, and cancers of the brain and skin.[143]

Cancer risks in slaughterhouse workers are of considerable interest, particularly, with regard to sarcomas, lymphomas, and leukemia's. However, relevant cancer studies of slaughterhouse workers have not been conducted until recently. The first such publication was the New Zealand case-control study of Smith et al. (1984), which found a relative risk of 2.8 (this is highly significant) for soft tissues sarcoma. Three more recent New Zealand case-control studies have found excess risks for non-Hodgkin's lymphoma, sarcomas and acute myeloid leukemia, while a United States study of slaughterhouse workers has found excess risks of Hodgkin's disease and cancer of other lymphatic tissue.

The high incidence of leukemia reported among persons living in areas where BLV is endemic (widespread) raises concern. Mortality from leukemia was significantly elevated among Wisconsin farmers residing in counties where dairying was prevalent.[144] A number of studies of other populations have been conducted. The most extensively studied group is farmers, which has shown an increased risk for many cancer sites, including Hodgkin's disease, leukemia, non-Hodgkin's lymphoma, and multiple myeloma. The similarity in patterns of risk for lymphatic and hemopoietic (blood and bone marrow) cancers in farmers and abattoir workers is particularly interesting, since common exposures may be involved.

Numerous reports of human leukemia clusters have been published showing a relationship between cattle or the dairy industry and the occurrence of human leukemia. A geographic correlation has been demonstrated in the Soviet Union, and Sweden between areas with a high frequency of bovine lymphosarcoma and high human leukemia rates. A Swedish case-control study, involving relatively small numbers, found that leukemia patients had BLV in their cattle herds more frequently than did neighborhood controls. In Iowa, Donham found a high positive correlation between the incidence of acute lymphatic leukemia (ALL) in males and cattle density, which was most striking for dairy cattle. Further, a 66% excess of cases of ALL was seen in those counties with large numbers of dairy cattle and BLV.[145]

A more recent case-control study by Donham examined

possible relationships between human ALL and exposure to dairy cattle and consumption of raw milk. However, the prevalence of antibodies to BLV in dairy herds to which the leukemia cases had been exposed was actually lower than that found in herds with which the controls had had contact.

BLV is a retrovirus. These retroviruses have been shown to cause tumors of the lymphatic and blood producing systems in all the higher nonhuman mammalian species studied to date. Slaughter house workers handling beef are potentially exposed to cancer viruses including the Bovine leukemia virus and statistically have a high risk for developing Hodgkin's disease and other cancers such as lymphosarcoma, reticulosarcoma and acute leukemia. The BLV virus has also been found in meat and unpasteurized milk. [146]

## ERADICATION OF BOVINE LEUKEMIA VIRUS

Dr. Caden, Germany, tested one herd of 286 Holstein-Friesen cattle every two weeks for four years to follow the spread of BLV infection. In this period the incidence of infection rose progressively from 4.8% to 52.6%.[147] This study shows that if no control measures for BLV are taken, an epidemic occurs. This is what is occurring in the United States.

The growing concern of many European and Latin American countries over the economic aspects of bovine leukemia infection is reflected by their implementation of eradication and/or control programs by the active role of their governments in these programs in supporting research on bovine leukemia. In the United States there are no federally sponsored control programs.[148] In many countries many herds are BLV free. It is feasible to achieve complete eradication provided the best methods of detecting BLV infection are used. [149] Some countries prohibit the importation of United States cattle, in view of the lack of an adequate testing program in the United States for bovine leukemia.[150]

## USDA FAILS TO ACT DUE TO POLITICS

The following was obtained from a symposium that was printed but not to be given to the public. However, I obtained it through the Freedom of Information Act.

At a bovine leukemia symposium sponsored by the United States Department of Agriculture[151] Dr. Marshak commented regarding eradication, "Well perhaps that isn't the correct word to use politically or economically these days. I think that we have got to stop being so sleepy about it. I know you in the Department of Agriculture can't decide these matters but I think that perhaps with pressure from the industry on the Department officials and the hierarchy and also through congress, we can perhaps get some legislation that will forward our goals in this problem. We are certainly not beginning to address them effectively at this point."

Mr. Mix also commented that "The dairyman is scared to death that he has a tumor condition in his herd and he therefore would probably object to a national program that would require culling and slaughter."[152]

Dr. Biel commented "In 1972 we did a survey for anaplasmosis. There was a concern about not wanting to have serums available that could be traced back to the herd of origin or that sort of thing—getting back to this business of confidentiality or what have you."

Dr. Marshak commented "We have been trying to talk to our people in Pennsylvania trying to explain, why don't we, on a herd to herd basis begin to clean up the disease. The reaction was, well, we do not want to talk about leukemia disease because it will scare the milk consumer so let's bury our heads and not do anything. So I think our Department of Agriculture—and I hate to say this because they are our hosts—have been sound asleep, and it won't be until the breeders and people in the cattle industry really get busy and press the right buttons that anything will happen. We can't do it; we've tried."

170

Dr. Nelson from the USDA: "But my only concern is that I don't want to leave any connotation or impression here that anybody's talking about an eradication program. Because that's a tough pill to swallow in many people's minds today. Now maybe down the road there will be such a thing, but at this point there isn't."

Dr. Marshak— "I think that we have to start thinking. If anything Mr. Mix said made any sense, this is an enormous threat to the American cattle industry, and I think that we have got to stop being so sleepy about it. I know you in the Department of Agriculture can't decide these matters, but I think that perhaps with pressure from the industry on the department officials and the hierarchy and also through the congress, we can perhaps get some legislation that will forward our goals in this problem. We certainly not beginning to address them effectively at this point."

Dr. Nelson, representing the United States Department of Agriculture commented, "I would like to be sure that the record is clear that we in the department have no intention of ever getting into an eradication program because that is a tough pill to swallow in many people's minds today."[153]

What a disgrace that because of this policy the American public has had to swallow milk contaminated with the Bovine leukemia virus.

### EARLY CONCLUSIONS SOLIDIFY

Before the new PCR test that has recently become available, human serological studies had all given results negative for antibodies to BLV. At that time the following conclusions were considered in the light of these negative data: 1) humans are not susceptible to infection with BLV, 2) the presently available techniques do not detect a serological response in humans, and 3) humans do not respond to BLV infection by producing serum. antibodies.[154]

Many attempts to identify antibodies to feline (cat) leukemia virus in humans had resulted in few positive samples, until a recent study demonstrated antibodies in 69% of 107 persons having contact with cats excreting feline leukemia virus. The study suggests that the positive results were due to increased sensitivity of serological techniques not available when the previous studies were conducted. A similar situation may partly explain why antibodies to the BLV have not been detected in humans. Now we know that humans have retrovirus in them from the PCR test and other antibody tests. Perhaps in the future we should act on our fears aroused by common sense, so that our health is not irrevocably damaged in the gap between suspicion and proof.

## PUBLIC HEALTH SIGNIFICANCE

Since other human viral pathogens are known to be transmitted through milk it is feasible that this could also be true for BLV. Milk-borne outbreaks have been caused by polio virus, and myxovirus, hepatitis virus, foot and mouth disease virus, (FMDV) and tick-borne encephalitis. Investigations have shown that milk can be a protective medium for these viruses. For example, FMDV, Maloney leukemia virus, Rauscher's leukemia virus and Rous sarcoma virus survive pasteurization.[155] We now know that we have retrovirus particles in the DNA of humans by the use of the Polymerase Chain Reaction Test which is 1000 times more accurate than other tests we had in the past to detect retrovirus.

Pasteurization appears therefore to render inactive many pathogenic viruses in milk; but there are disquieting exceptions. Reassessment of techniques used and further data are required.[156] Considering the foregoing non-dairy milk would be the safest milk to drink. Using dairy milk in cooking would also be safer than pasteurized milk.

There is every reason to expect that viruses pathogenic to man, permitted to contaminate various raw food materials, would survive many of today's accepted processing and reconstitution regimens. The viruses generally are more resistant than the vegetative cells of bacteria to adverse conditions. Yet many of our major food preservation practices were developed largely on the basis of bacterial control.[157]

## WAS A SCIENTIST BOYCOTTED?

A personal letter from Jorge F. Ferrer MD, who is section chief of Viral Oncology at the University of Pennsylvania stated the following to me. "As you know, both NIH and the USDA have continued to dismiss the potential public health significance of BLV. The argument given is that there is no direct evidence that BLV infects humans. This argument, however, ignores the fact that the studies conducted thus far on this question are fragmentary and incomplete, and do not rule out the possibility that BLV, a BLV variant or a closely related virus may infect humans." Later on Dr. Ferrer says: "I believe that the first recommendation in regard to the potential public health significance of BLV should be to conduct the studies that are required to critically evaluate whether or not BLV can infect humans. Neither NIH nor the USDA seem to be interested in providing financial support for these studies. At least all our attempts to obtain this support have been unsuccessful despite the fact that because of the expertise of its staff and the resources available, our Unit has been in an exceptionally favorable position to conduct the needed research." [158]

### DELANEY AMENDMENT

The Delaney Amendment was passed in Congress to prevent cancer. What did the consumer want the Delaney Amendment to accomplish? If a substance caused cancer in animals it would be illegal to be added to foods. We can surmise that the American consumer wants the Department of Agriculture to do everything it can to eliminate BLV in an eradication program to reduce BLV in cattle. If BLV can cause cancer in cows and other animals, then the cows and milk are not healthy and should be eliminated. Pasteurized milk can be contaminated with raw milk as we well know in Chicago in 1985. BLV poses a much serious problem than TB. or Brucellosis. It is hard to understand why the Delaney

Amendment was not used to  include milk that contained the BLV virus and also caused cancer in animals.

### GRANT APPROVAL:

I submitted a grant proposal on milk consumption and its relationship to leukemia in Oct. 1982. My recommendations were approved for 300,000 dollars with a priority score of 377. However, I was not funded because the budget was cut in Congress. The following was their final critique detailing their concerns:

"While there is some plausibility to the hypothesis that the investigators have raised, it is unlikely that the present study will have much ability to evaluate it. If the investigators concern that the bovine leukemia virus is not inactivated (with respect to cancer causation) by pasteurization, then effectively everyone in their study population will be exposed to the virus, and no discrimination of exposed and nonexposed individuals will be possible. If, on the other hand, the bovine leukemia virus is inactivated by pasteurization, the study will still have difficulty: (a) the exposure of the population to unpasteurized cheese (e.g., Swiss or blue cheese) is widespread; (b) many of the respondents will be unsure as to the pasteurization status of the cheese they have eaten in the past; and  the frequency of ingestion of raw milk may be low (it is not documented by the investigators), although it is being marketed in California."

What the reviews of the grant proposal were saying was that since nearly everyone drinks milk and eats cheese, it is impossible to get a control group of people that have not drunk milk most of their lifetime so an epidemiology study would be nearly impossible to do. Therefore, we as consumers must use our common sense as to whether we will drink milk and eat dairy products. When the dairy industry sees that the consumer seriously wants healthy milk from healthy cows, it will promote an eradication program of the Bovine leukemia virus as the industry is interested in healthy profits. Dairy products are in most foods we buy today. Look at the label on foods.

Most products will contain whey, casein, cheese, milk, or butter. Even in health food stores most diet supplements, protein supplements, nutritional supplements contain whey or casein.

## DIET AND CANCER

In the spotlight of carrying an excess risk of cancer is the diet heaped with tender well-marbled steaks, heavily smoked and salt cured foods, rich ice creams and other high fat dairy products such as cheddar cheese—all washed down with too much beer, wine and whisky. The anti-cancer diet is high in fruit, vegetables and whole grain cereals. The Committee on Diet, Nutrition and Cancer Guidelines called on Americans to eat less fat. It was against fats that the panel found the strongest scientific evidence of an association with certain cancers.[159] It is my feeling that fats are a confounder, meaning not the real cause of cancer, but that it is most likely the retroviruses that are responsible for causing cancer.

## POTENTIAL HAZARD OF BLV TO MAN

The last and most crucial question remains: Is BLV a threat to humans? Since BLV is so widespread, epidemiology studies are not feasible, but common sense requires us to consider BLV in light of the Delaney act which states that any substance added to food and causes cancer in animals should be presumed to be able to cause cancer in humans.

## RECOMMENDATIONS ON RAW MILK

Present technology cannot produce any raw milk, certified or otherwise, that can be assured free of human pathogens. Accordingly, the US Animal Health Association, the National Association of State Public Health Veterinarians, the Conference of State and Territorial Epidemiologists, and the American Academy of Pediatrics have adopted policy statements advocating milk for human consumption should be pasteurized. On July 20, 1980, the House of Delegates of the American Veterinary Medical Association passed a resolution that only pasteurized milk products should be sold for human consumption. They further resolved that in those states where the sale of unpasteurized milk is authorized, those products should be labeled "Not pasteurized and may contain organisms that cause human disease."[160] In spite of these resolutions several states allow raw milk to be sold. An example is my own state, Oregon.

## CHEESE

Cheeses commonly made from unpasteurized milk require minimum aging of 60 to 90 days in the United States and certain other countries as a safety measure against survival of pathogenic bacteria. The efficacy of this requirement against viral agents has not been adequately explored. Once introduced, polio virus and other enteric viruses have been found to persist in cottage cheese curd, cheddar cheese and sour milk products.

Present technology cannot produce any raw milk or raw aged cheese that can be free of Human Pathogens. The exposure of the U.S. population to unpasteurized cheese (e.g., Swiss or blue cheese) is widespread, and these cheeses may contain BLV even after the aging process. [161] [162] Always look for "Made from Pasteurized Milk" on labels when buying cheese.

## CHILDREN WANT MILK FREE OF LEUKEMIA

Our goal is to serve to our children and adults, milk free of leukemia virus produced from leukemia free cows. Pasteurization of milk and cheese should be promoted and an eradication program of bovine leukemia virus in dairy cattle in the United States should be encouraged. An eradication program for BLV would not be costly for dairymen. It could be easily be accomplished in 2-3 years. There would be savings in medical costs as it would lower the cost of Medicare and this would help balance the United States budget since retroviruses are associated with human cancer. We must do all that we can to get our government and the dairy industry to improve our milk supply. We require milk from healthy cows. Lloyd states that

176

until the question is totally resolved regarding a human hazard from BLV, recommendations are to drink pasteurized milk and abstain from eating raw meat.[163]

## ERADICATION AND CONTROL PROGRAMS

Many European Countries have eradication and control programs for BLV. Some countries prohibit the importation of United States cattle, in view of the lack of an adequate testing program in the United States for bovine leucosis.[164] Switzerland has no infected BLV cattle. Other countries have reduced their infection down to 1-2%. The United States Animal Health Association adopted a resolution recommending that the animal and Plant Health Inspection Service of USDA institute a voluntary program for the establishment and maintenance of BLV free herds. The proposal was presented to the USDA. The USDA has never responded to it; so there was no regulatory activity of any kind until recently. Even now, all we have is a limited voluntary program enacted with the States in charge of the program. Many foreign countries have successful eradication and/or control programs for BLV.[165]

## A MENU OF DISEASES

A paper published gave results indirectly suggesting that retroviruses with similar properties could cause various brain and nerve diseases in man. Recently it was reported that in some patients with multiple sclerosis an antibody was detected which cross reacted with human T-cell viruses, and the cells of the cerebrospinal fluid contained retroviral RNA that was related to but distinct from human viruses. It was found that the BLV genome could be easily transmitted by co-cultivation of virus-productive sheep cells to human malignant glioma cell lines, to neuroblastoma cells of human malignant glioma cell lines, to neuroblastoma cells of human origin, as well as to rat glioma cells. Therefore, cells of brain and nerve origin are considered susceptible to BLV infection and replication. The results confirm indirectly the recent suggestions that leukemia virus or similar retroviruses of this type could be involved in the process which leads to multiple sclerosis.[166] I can add to this concern because, of the 10 patients I have taken care of with multiple sclerosis, all had drunk raw milk in their lifetimes.

Potentially, bovine leukemia virus seems to be a broader infectious agent than originally anticipated. The virus could be easily spread by milk from infected cows. It seems to be inactivated by effective pasteurization but lymphocytes from infected animals are frequently present in milk. The virus transmission by infected cells is more effective than by the virus itself. In chimpanzees leukemia induced by milk from cows shedding BLV was also reported. [167] Antibodies to BLV are present in pasteurized milk.

Other countries have eliminated BLV or bovine Lymphosarcoma by eradication programs. We have not. We expect pasteurization to kill all pathogens. It won't. Pasteurization kills only 99.9% of all pathogenic bacteria or 2 Standard deviations found in the raw milk. Milk should come from healthy cows for pasteurization, not cows with BIV or BLV.

After the milk is produced on the dairy farm it is mixed in large vats so it is no longer possible to spot bloody milk now. When the cow is being milked with a milking machine, frequently blood vessels break in the udder of the cow. There may be a fissure in one of the teats that allows the bleeding. When milk was in 10 gallon milk cans it could be condemned as being bloody like a strawberry milk shake.

Aids can be transmitted by blood in humans. Cows have Bovine AIDS. Milk contains blood and blood cells. The Human Aids Virus, The Cow Aids virus, the Bovine leukemia virus are all retroviruses and have similar properties. Pasteurized milk was accidentally contaminated with raw milk in one of the worst salmonella-related dairy disaster in April 1985, in the Chicago area. 180,000 illnesses were linked to the outbreak. This pasteurized milk which people drank would also have been contaminated with BIV and BLV.

# GRAVEST PUBLIC HEALTH THREAT OF THE CENTURY

At a USAHA meeting one researcher reported that Bovine leukemia virus in the United States is one of the gravest public health threats of the century. One would think that in our health-conscious societies, we would be doing everything in our power to stop the spread of this disease, but we are not. The same population that threw out its muffin mix two-and-a-half years ago because of the purely hypothetical risk posed by trace residues of the pesticide EDB seems oddly blasé about BLV. Even with scientists and researchers asking for eradication programs the beef and dairy industries have influenced the USDA and FDA not to allow it. So we get cancer, and our children get leukemia. It is urgent that we now shift from relative complacency to action in preventing the future spread of BLV in dairy cattle. We can begin by discarding those naive assumptions and simplistic solutions which to date have so hampered any aggressive preventive medicine policy.

## NAVAJO INDIANS

Dr. Gibbons, a medical doctor and former medical editor of the Saturday Evening Post, read my article in Health and Healing and was inspired to write the book  why the Navajo Indians never get cancer. In an interview with Dr. Gibbons that was published in the Journal Alexandria, in Virginia on July 11, 1983. He said, "There's no doubt in my mind, that eggs and milk spread cancer. I've watched 5,000 Indians for 17 years with not one case of breast cancer. There's something the Indians are doing right that whites aren't. I've come to the conclusion that Indians don't eat eggs and they don't drink milk. It's not in their diet".

Gibbons believes that most forms of cancer are caused by a virus. "Chickens and cows often suffer from virus-caused cancer," he said, "and the animals' virus are passed on to humans by eating eggs, drinking milk and eating red meat. If you don't cook the egg, you're eating the virus. Until recently we

179

ate raw eggs all the time—in ice cream, mayonnaise, eggnog. Milk has the same problem. Pasteurization helps, but it probably is not adequate. The temperature they use when they pasteurize milk isn't hot enough or long enough to kill the virus."

In the infected lymphocytes, BLV is integrated with chromosomal DNA in the form of a provirus in a small number of copies per genome. BLV remains latent (asleep) and viremia is not observed in the infected animal. However, although replication is undetectable, the antibodies appear in the infected animals but who are unable to eliminate the virus, and the animals remain carriers till the end of their lives. Therefore, diagnosis of bovine leukemia is usually based on detection of specific antibodies. However, the lack of serological response is not tantamount to the lack of infection, since only the presence of provirus DNA integrated with the cell genome can serve as an unquestionable criterion. [168] The USDA refuses to check milk and meat for these antibodies of BIV and BLV because they do not want the public to know about it.

On Feb. 24, 1987 a letter to Mark O. Hatfield, United States Senator from the Food and Drug Administration by Hugh C. Cannon stated. 'This is in reply to the letter of January 29, 1987, on behalf of Virgil M. Hulse, M.D. Dr. Hulse is concerned about Bovine leukemia virus and its potential cancer hazard to humans. The Food and Drug Administration has given this subject much thought over the years since the Bovine leukemia virus' discovery in 1969. There remain many unanswered questions concerning its transmissibility, infectivity, and pathogenicity in humans. Please be assured that the Agency will also give much thought to the health hazard potential of the Bovine leukemia virus in its consideration of this significant issue."

# LETTER SENT TO THE UNITED STATES ANIMAL HEALTH ASSOCIATION

I was not able to attend the meeting of the United States Animal Health Association in Nov. 3, 1992 of which I am a member. I sent the members a letter urging them to institute a compulsory eradication program for the Bovine leukemia virus. Instituting this program would help insure the American public that we are receiving milk from healthy, leukemia- free cows. This letter included much of what I have discussed in this chapter. I briefly reiterated the different studies done in the U.S., Denmark, and Sweden. I cited the close correlation between prevalence of BLV in cattle and the incidence of leukemia and other cancers in human population. I commended the great success of Switzerland, Germany and France in eradicating BLV in their herds, suggesting that we could be as successful in cleaning up our herds. I told that that I am on the Board of Health for Jackson County, in Oregon. We have gallons of raw milk sold in nearly every store in our county. We have been unsuccessful in enacting a compulsory pasteurization requirement in the State of Oregon. We certainly need help from the United States government. Just this last week a patient came into me stating it was recommended that the members of her Health and exercise club drink raw milk. Another friend told me that in a day care center for children that the caregiver and her children drank raw milk. We have a large Mexican population in our area who do not read English and could accidentally pick up the raw milk in our supermarkets. For those that drink raw milk there would be less BLV in raw milk if we had a eradication program for BLV in dairy cows. It was disappointing to me that the committee did not recommend an eradication program and the following year they did not recommend the dairies that sell raw milk should be BLV free. I felt indebted to the Dairy Industry for a $1000 dollar Bob Hope Scholarship the California Dairy Industry Board awarded me to attend Cal Poly where I received my BS degree in Dairy Manufacturing, but my last hope to work through the dairy establishment and the government had been shattered. I then determined to write a book to bring it to the attention of the United States consumer. It was my goal in writing the letter, and it remains my goal in writing this book, for America to produce milk free of retroviruses from healthy BLV-free herds.

## SUMMARY

I have tried during my lifetime, without success, to influence the dairy industry to clean up the milk supply. Because of my inability to get an eradication program enacted from the USDA, the FDA, through Congress or through the Dairy Industry, I decided I would have to take my case to the American public.

In my family practice it has been distressing to see my patients developing cancer and dying. My wife and I took care of my mother when she died of cancer. My oldest son died of cancer. If you have buried a loved one you understand. I am not anti-milk. I am not anti-beef. I just want this country to be more concerned with producing clean milk and beef from healthy cows. We are not doing our best; we can do better. Nothing is more important than our children. I held my first baby 47 years ago. He was a beautiful baby boy. Now he is dead from cancer. I hope that this book will prevent this from happening to your children. What do you want for your kids? They deserve the best. I have a dream that we can stop this epidemic of cancer by improving our milk and food supply. Let us make the United States a healthier place to live. We can do it.

It took me nearly 35 years to find it was useless to get the dairy industry to have an eradication program for BLV. Harold Lyman had gone to Washington DC for over 2 years trying to lobby and get reform. He stated you need to lobby with large sums of money to get anything done, this is why this book had to be written. My intent is to give the American public the facts they deserve. Only the dairy industry or our government can decide to enact an eradication program. Such a program will only be put into place when consumers stop eating dairy products and drinking milk that they cannot trust; then the dairy industry will listen. Decide now, with the information about the dangers of BLV, what you and your family will do.

The epidemic of Bovine leukemia virus is increasing with lightening speed. The cows are giving off the Bovine leukemia virus in their milk and America's men, women and children are drinking milk every day with this retrovirus. The proviral DNA loves to mutate and hide and then cause cancer in the cows. In all likelihood the same thing is happening in people. We are reminded of the recent abominable practice of feeding dead cancerous cows back to cows and with this change in cows from being a herbivorous animal to a cannibal that disastrous consequences will occur. We are on the brink of new infectious disease epidemics and we can predict that in the future this will be dangerous to us all. In a previous chapter in this book you read about the Mad Cow Disease, one more consequence of feeding cows to cows. We must learn our lessons and not let this happen again. We should not play with fire. I believe that by informing others of the dangers of dairy consumption: cancer is combated, and health is promoted.

The Bovine leukemia virus is unpredictable. We do not know what it has done in the past. We do not know what it might do in the future. We do not know bovine leukemia's function and structure or how it mutates and causes cancer in cows. It could be mutating even today and causing cancer in humans. Many people are skeptical when considering whether the Bovine leukemia virus can cause problems in humans. However, when we are feeding sheep and cows and other dead animals to cows, we are providing a perfect setup for an outbreak of a virus that can jump species. This is a natural laboratory for rapid virus evolution. Continuance of such disgraceful practices within the beef and dairy industries bears ghastly implications for the human race

## WHAT CAN YOU DO

Please write to your State and US congressman regarding the urgent need to: 1. Serve our children and adults milk free of leukemia virus produced from leukemia free cows. 2. Eradicate BLV in dairy cattle in the US is imperative to obtain milk from healthy cows. 3. Stop feeding dead diseased cows to cows to increase milk production    4. Use your common sense as to what milk you are willing to purchase and drink.

# CHAPTER FIVE

# COW AIDS

Yes, AIDS in Cows! Retroviruses, so much in the news these days, are particularly dangerous because they can work backwards from the usual flow of genetic information, and pervert the very code of existence of a cell. Here is an example of how retroviruses work. BLV, as all other retroviruses, does the following upon entering a cell. With the action of Reverse trancriptase (an enzyme) it is changed to a double stranded viral DNA. The double-stranded viral DNA, known as the provirus, is transported to the nucleus where it integrates into the host chromosomes and becomes part of the DNA of the animal. The virus is then a permanent part of the cell, and the provirus is replicated every time the cell divides. The provirus can remain in the latent (asleep), or unexpressed state (not producing virus) in an individual cell, although there is probably active multiplication occurring in infected cells somewhere in the body continuously.

## COW AIDS VIRUS RELATED TO HUMAN AIDS VIRUS

The USDA National Animal Disease Center in Ames, Iowa, in recent years reported that a new virus is widely distributed among United States cattle and seems to be prevalent among dairy cattle in the South. The virus is called "bovine immunodeficiency virus" (BIV), because its structure and other characteristics are closely related to HIV, the human AIDS virus. The virus was subsequently found to have genes, antibodies and a structure that was similar to the human immunodeficiency virus. Preliminary research results indicate that the virus may impair the immune systems of cattle just as the AIDS virus does in patients with the acquired immune deficiency syndrome and hasten death.

## INFECTS MANY DIFFERENT ANIMAL SPECIES

Lentiviruses are a type of retrovirus of which BIV in cattle is one. Others exist in some sheep, horses, cats, goats, monkeys and humans (the human AIDS virus). Each of these viruses causes a chronic, insidious, and frequently lethal disease in its respective host. [169]

## CAUSES ENLARGED LYMPH NODES

The USDA has also been able to transfer infection among goats, sheep, and rabbits by blood transfer. Increased numbers of lymphocytes in the blood (similar to what occurs in leukemia) and enlarged lymph nodes under the skin have been seen in some animals. Dairy herd records indicated that animals were being culled because of health problems and that the incidence of lymphosarcoma (cancer) was quite high. Serological (antibody) tests for BIV, bovine leukemia virus, and bovine syncytial virus proved that infections with all three of these bovine retroviruses were represented in single herds and sometimes all three infect the same cow at the same time. Blood studies identified elevated white blood cells, primarily lymphocytes, in these cows.

## DISCOVERY

BIV was first isolated in domestic cattle in the 1970s, and is called bovine immunodeficiency virus (BIV) because its genetic structure is so closely related to the Human Immunodeficiency Virus (HIV) or AIDS virus. Scientists have successfully infected human cells with BIV, and at least one study suggested that BIV may play a role in either malignant or slow viruses in man. This virus was isolated and reported by Van Der Maaten in 1972 and was placed in Nitrogen storage for years and nearly forgotten about, but it did not draw attention since, at that time, most efforts were directed towards research on the Bovine leukemia virus. However, new interest was shown on the Bovine Immunodeficiency Virus (BIV), because of the urgent need for developing animal models for the acquired immunodeficiency syndrome (AIDS) after it was discovered.

Bovine immunodeficiency virus had been isolated only once for the virus to actually grow in cell culture in the laboratory, and all attempts to obtain additional isolates had failed except recently it was isolated from an infected rabbits spleen. Now it has been recovered from the leucocytes of cattle infected with the BLV, including cows with enlarged lymph nodes, lesions in the brain and spinal cord, progressive weakness, losing weight, and wasting away.

## BIV CAUSES DISEASE IN THE BRAIN

In the South, the average frequency within individual herds can be considerably higher. For example, average frequencies of 40% in beef and 64% in dairy herds were found in the Louisiana area; and, notably, many of these BIV-positive animals were infected with Bovine leukemia virus (BLV). The virus prefers to multiply and cause disease in the immune system and the brain. In herds, cows have shown a viral meningoencephalitis (infection of the brain). [170] It has been observed that cows with a marked increase of white blood cells in high-producing dairy herds, seem to have an increased incidence of bovine cancer.[171] Although cattle are the natural host of BIV, BIV can infect other animals such as rabbits, sheep and goats. BIV has been isolated from a spleen of BIV-infected rabbits.[172]

The isolation of two pathogenic retroviruses from cattle, BLV and BIV, related respectively to the only known human retroviruses, HTLV-1, HTLV-2, and HIV, caused concern that these two viruses working together causes more cancer in cows than if the cows were infected with only one of the Retroviruses. There is also concern that they may be promoting human diseases such as cancer? Is BIV in cattle a problem that has gone undiagnosed or misdiagnosed due to the overriding presence of other viruses, such as BLV which also causes lymphocytosis (increased white blood cells)? It was thought that this may be the case, and in some instances BLV may occur as a secondary infection in BIV-infected animals, much as HTLV-

I does in AIDS patients. [173]

## EPIDEMIC OF COW AIDS IN BRITAIN

An outbreak of bovine AIDS in Britain was reported recently in cows. These cows showed a wide range of obvious clinical spectra including nerve degeneration, weight loss, mouth ulcers, and respiratory infections.. [174]

Millions of cattle are produced in the world every year, but only a very small sample of cows has been analyzed for BIV infection. Surveys that have been done revealed a seroprevalence of 40% in beef herds and 64% in dairy herds (ranges, 5-53% in beef and 37-82% in dairy herds).[175]

## BIV COWS MAY NOT LOOK SICK

Control of BIV infection in the U.S. has not been actively pursued due to the presumably innocuous clinical course following experimental inoculation of animals in a short time. Usually the dairy cows are culled and slaughtered before the infection has reached its full blown disease potential in the cow. In cows, disease obvious by observation may require long incubation periods to occur. [176] Lentiviruses of which BIV and HIV are a member produce debilitating diseases which may last from months to years following initial infection. Factors which may increase the expression of the retrovirus genome from its latent (sleepy) state in vivo (life), thereby resulting in disease, include co-infection with other viruses, such as herpesviruses, and nonspecific antigenic stimulation such as infection, age, and pesticides. Preliminary research results indicate that the virus may impair the immune systems of cattle, just as the AIDS virus does in patients with the acquired immune deficiency syndrome.

The USDA Animal and Plant Health Inspection Service, working with the National Institutes of Health, has been quietly engaged in investigating the potential links between BIV and human disease since 1987. Bovine immunodeficiency virus (BIV) is a Retrovirus but different from the bovine leukemia

188

virus. When BIV was inoculated in calves, the calves developed fever and changes in the number of white blood cells in blood, mainly lymphocytes. It caused the lymph nodes to enlarge. The BIV was originally isolated from animals with a increased white blood cells and enlarged lymph nodes. It did not seem to cause cancer by itself.

## CROSS REACTION WITH HUMAN AIDS VIRUS

Six human sera that showed strong reactions against HIV-1 cross reacted with BIV. This is the first report of human sera with antibody to BIV. The cross-reactivity likely represent reactivity to genes found on BIV and HIV since humans at risk for BIV have not readily been shown to show antibodies to BIV infection. Since BIV can infect a variety of bovine and other nonhuman cells in tissue culture, it is important to ensure that cultured cells used as sources of biologicals for humans be screened for BIV infection. [177]

## INFECTIONS RISING IN HUMANS

Interestingly infections have moved up to third place in all causes of deaths in humans. This should behoove us to do all we can to prevent infecting our bodies by watching to see that what we eat is not loaded with viruses and bacteria. Disturbing is the fact that Fetal bovine sera used at least in the past in preparation of bovine and human biologicals such as medicine and blood products have shown that a variety of bovine viruses were present in about 30% of fetal bovine sera.

## COWS AIDS VIRUS SPREADING IN U.S.

Meanwhile the cow AIDS virus is continuing to spread among American cattle with no cure in sight. The economic impact of BIV on the beef and dairy industries is likely to be devastating in the years to come as more and more cattle become infected with cow AIDS and succumb to a range of opportunistic and parasitic diseases stemming from weakened immune systems.

189

## LENTIVIRUS CAUSES ARTHRITIS AND BRAIN DISEASE

The Lentiviruses are associated with inflammatory diseases (example arthritis) and immunodeficiencies (like AIDS). Lentivirus disease is slow in onset, often involves multiple organs, and is severely, debilitating, although not always fatal. As examples HIV I in man and some strains of simian immunodeficiency viruses in monkeys induce a fatal immunodeficiency syndrome and encephalopathy (brain disease). In contrast, caprine arthritis encephalitis virus in goats induces a chronic arthritis, encephalitis, and mastitis without significant mortality. The mechanism(s) by which each of the pathogenic lentiviruses induce disease is not clearly understood but certainly is related to the interaction of virus with host immune cells.

Persistent lymphadenopathy (enlarged lymph nodes and glands) and central nervous system lesions are common features of Lentivirus infections. In BIV-infected cattle, the brain lesions are suggestive of a viral encephalitis when examined under a microscope. BIV DNA has been demonstrated in lymph nodes and brains of infected cattle by the Polymerase Chain Reaction test.

## USDA REFUSES TO CHECK MILK FOR BIV ANTIBODIES

It is now known that while a Lentivirus may remain transcriptionally silent (asleep or hiding) in an infected cell until appropriate endogenous or exogenous factors activate the virus, the infection in the animal is never truly latent (asleep), as active virus production is probably occurring somewhere in the body. Eventually the animal succumbs to the accumulated effects of low-level replication (virus production), and obvious disease results.[178]

Despite increasing anecdotal (circumstantial) evidence linking bovine leukemia virus and bovine immunodeficiency virus to potential human health risks, the USDA has steadfastly refused to check slaughtered meat, milk, and dairy products to see if they contain antibodies to these retroviruses. It seems that they just do not want to scare the milk consumer. Every day, Americans consume beef and dairy products from cows, some of which are infected with bovine leukemia virus and cow AIDS virus, without any assurance that the products are safe.

It is shocking that the human AIDS virus and BLV can be activated by other viruses such as the herpesviruses, and that other factors may also activate retroviruses, such as continual antigenic stimulation.[179]

## IMMUNOSUPRESSION DIFFICULT TO RECOGNIZE

It must be recognized that a mild or borderline immunosupression is very difficult to recognize in dairy herds because animals with decreased immune function from BIV would probably be dropping out of infected herds for the same reasons that they have always been removed—only at a higher rate of slaughter due to decreased milk production and high somatic cell counts (blood cells) in milk, usually lymphocytes.[180] Remember that BLV and BIV, are related respectively to the only known human retroviruses, HTLV-1(causes Human T-cell leukemia and widespread in Japan). HTLV-II (causes Hairy-cell leukemia) and HIV(causes human AIDS).

## NO CURE FOR BOVINE AIDS VIRUS

Government researchers say that the virus poses no threat to human health. Jeremy Rifkin of the Foundation on Economic Trends a watch dog group says that infected cattle should not be sent to slaughter any more, and they should not be milked until long-term studies can be done. That the USDA should set up emergency protocol to start locating every infected cow in the United States and isolate them and I agree with him. There is no cure for BIV.

In a formal response to a petition submitted by the Foundation on Economic Trends, Dr. James Wyngaarden, at that time the director of the NIH, and Bert Hawkins, administrator of the Animal and Plant Health Inspection Service, reported that "cattle sera from herds in different localities in the U.S. are being collected to screen for BIV infection." The agency directors also announced that they were in the process of developing "sensitive assays to screen human sera of individuals at some risk of exposure to the virus, either through occupation or some other means." [181]

## BOVINE AIDS VIRUS SUPPRESSES THE IMMUNE SYSTEM

Then in 1991 the USDA released the results of its four-year investigation on BIV to Jeremy Rifkin of the Foundation on Economic Trends. The findings were disturbing. According to the USDA, the cow AIDS virus is widespread among dairy cows and beef cattle and is suspected of suppressing the animals' immune systems, making them susceptible to a wide range of diseases, including mastitis (infected udder) and cancer. The USDA says that it does not yet know "whether exposure to BIV proteins causes human sera to...become HIV positive." The USDA is continuing its investigations.

## BLOODY MILK

As we know Aids can be transmitted by contaminated blood in humans. Cows have Bovine AIDS. Milk contains blood and blood cells. As other milk inspectors have, I have condemned daily hundreds of pounds of bloody milk working for the State of California. That was in the days when milk was delivered in 10 gallon cans. Now bloody milk is mixed with other milk in the large milk holding tanks and it no longer looks bloody. But the blood is still there, now it is merely diluted with all the other milk from the milking herd. If the udder of a single cow was bloody and it was pumped into the milk tank the milk would still be contaminated even thought it would appear white due to the dilution factor.

## IS IT SAFE TO CONSUME DAIRY PRODUCTS?

The AIDS Virus, The Cow AIDS virus, the Bovine leukemia virus are all Retro viruses and have similar properties. Other countries have eliminated BLV or bovine Lymphosarcoma by eradication programs. We have not. We expect pasteurization to kill all pathogens. It will not. Pasteurization kills only 99.9% of all pathogenic bacteria or 2 standard deviations (a statistical term) found in the raw milk. In fact, pasteurized milk was accidentally contaminated with raw milk in one of the worst ever salmonella-related dairy disasters in the Chicago during April 1985, resulting in 180,000 illnesses that were linked to the outbreak. This pasteurized milk which people drank would also have been contaminated with BIV and BLV. Milk should come from healthy cows to be pasteurized, not cows with BIV or BLV. Reader draw your own conclusions, make up your own mind if you believe it is safe to consume dairy products at this time.

## HOW PREVALENT IS BIV

A recent study reported in the Veterinary Microbiology found that a 38% of all of the cows in the herd were infected with BLV. In one herd and another herd at Mississippi State University 58% of all the cows in the herd were infected with BIV. A cumulative BIV seroprevalence (of all herds examined) of 50% was found in the Mississippi animals. BIV infection may be common in both beef and dairy cattle. One herd had a 64% incidence of BIV in a dairy herd with a high incidence of lymphosarcoma, lymphadenopathy, and persistent health problems, and in addition 74% of this herd was positive for Bovine leukemia virus (BLV). BIV was reported in 40% in beef herds and 64% in dairy herds was detected in Louisiana cattle. All of these studies provide further evidence that BIV infection is widespread among animals in the southern United States. Additionally, insect transmission of equine (horse) infectious anemia virus was reported. It is believed that BIV may also be spread by blood sucking insects. The incidence of BIV infection in the northern United States where biting insects are

193

fewer is quite low, lending support to the important role of insects in the transmission of BIV. [182] This is compelling information that should require our government to act quickly to protect the U.S. population from this cow AIDS virus.

## SUMMARY

Since it was learned that BIV is widely distributed among U.S. cattle and seems to be prevalent among dairy cattle in the South. BIV has been successfully isolated from the spleen of experimentally infected rabbits. We have also been able to transfer infection among goats and sheep by blood transfer. Persistent lymphocytosis and enlarged subcutaneous hemolymph nodes have been seen in some animals. Limited blood studies have, as stated above, provided evidence that BIV infections are widely distributed among U.S. cattle. In two herds that were good producers and well cared for it was noted that variable peaks and valleys in numbers were reported in both herds when sent to the slaughter house. Herd records indicated that animals were being culled because of health problems and that the incidence of lymphosarcoma was quite high. Serological tests for BIV, bovine leukemia virus, and bovine syncytial virus, another retrovirus, provided proof that infections with all three of these bovine retroviruses were represented in herds, and hematological studies identified elevated white blood cells, primarily to lymphocytes in these cows.

It is unlikely that the viruses identified to date represent all of the retroviruses responsible for human disease. Lymphatic disorders in general, and immunodeficiencies in particular, merit closer scrutiny for a retroviral etiologic agent. Then there are other diseases that medical science has not been able to find the responsible cause. Many scientists believe that these diseases with unknown causes may well be caused by retroviruses.

## ERADICATION

We should get a recommendation for a compulsory eradication program for BLV such as that which has been implemented in other countries, and for BIV; but so far no such recommendation has been forthcoming. Many doctors and health professionals believe we will see a reduction in all types of cancer in humans, especially those cancers in humans related to fat consumption, when we wipe out BIV and BLV in cattle. Although not proven there is considerable evidence that it is the Retroviruses from animal sources rather than the fat itself that is the reason for many human cancers such as breast, colon, prostrate cancer, lymphomas and leukemia. Epidemiology studies done in China, where populations eat little meat or dairy products, amazingly have very little cancer, osteoporosis, or heart disease.

### WHAT CAN YOU DO?

Until the United States Department of Agriculture institutes a compulsory eradication program for Bovine leukemia virus and Bovine immunodeficiencey Virus that will insure the American Public that we are receiving milk from healthy cows free of leukemia, cancer and AIDS, my family and I are going to drink nondairy milk that is fortified with calcium and that does not contain sodium caseinate, and whey, which are by-products of cows' milk. But you must decide what you are going to do after considering all the facts. I hope you make the right decision.

# CHAPTER SIX

# RETROVIRUSES

## NEW FROM THE NATIONAL INSTITUTES OF HEALTH

In the last 10 years new retroviruses have been emerging with increasing frequency (many of which were previously thought to be incapable of infecting humans) as disease-causing agents. We now know that retrovirus particles can cause cancer by recombining with the DNA of the human or animal cell in which they have become infected.

They can insert their DNA code into the human or animal they infect by an enzymatic process called Reverse Transcription. This cell will then reproduce itself according to its new, mutated DNA. The resulting daughter cells can be latent (sleeping) in the body for years before they are expressed as cancer or AIDS. It has been shown that the human AIDS virus directly causes cancer. Dr. McGrath reported in Cancer Research that the AIDS virus inserted its genetic material into a cell's DNA, and apparently switched on a nearby cancer-causing gene, starting up a less common variety of lymphoma called non B-cell lymphoma. Researchers say, after considering the data, that as many as a third of non-B-cell lymphomas in AIDS patients may be directly caused by the virus.

Eric Johnson from the National Institute of Health[183] reported that a variety of retroviruses are highly prevalent in chickens and turkeys and cause tumors in them. Commercial chickens are positive for antibodies, and a proportion actually carry infectious viruses. Retroviruses may be present in chicken products and in eggs, thus human exposure is virtually universal. Most, but not all of the blood studies in humans have been negative. Given the known behavior of these retroviruses in mammals, this was not unexpected. Just because humans may not have an antibody reaction to a retrovirus does not mean that they have not been infected. In an overwhelming majority of cases there is evidence that tumor induction can occur in the absence of virological and serological evidence of infection. This means no antibodies can be detected in the blood of the person infected.

Poultry retroviruses have been shown to be strong cancer producing agents. A single virus particle can be sufficient to change a healthy cell to one that is cancerous. There is some epidemiological evidence associating poultry exposure with cancer in humans. Again, antibodies can be absent, even in the presence of viral reproduction within tumors. These observations are important in assessing whether retroviruses can cause cancer in humans. Yet the mechanisms involved are poorly understood. The link between chicken retroviruses and mammal or human cancer is incomplete. With the knowledge that humans are universally exposed to these retroviruses, and the fact that some of these retroviruses could be causing cancer; knowing for certain whether these retroviruses can cause cancer in humans becomes imperative.

Johnson states that if we can detect these retroviruses in human tumor cells with the polymerase chain reaction (PCA) more than often in tumor cells than those humans without cancer, it would provide definitive evidence of a casual association. There is an urgent need now for these types of studies to be undertaken.

RNA retroviruses mutate frequently because sometimes the copying of these large pieces of RNA becomes very sloppy. One RNA piece might cross over to another, mixing up their genes. Results are that during viral replication (inserting RNA into DNA in the cell), they often mix their proteins and sometimes even their genes in several different ways. They may mutate by making erroneous substitutions of some of their nucleotides (parts of RNA genes) partly due to mistakes made by the enzyme reverse transcriptase during DNA synthesis. Reverse transcriptase is an enzyme that the RNA virus uses to transfer its gene information into the cell of the animal it is infecting. During this process pieces of their genetic information may be lost. Note that the conversion of a retrovirus from RNA to DNA occurs only inside the cell. Such an arrangement is most likely due to the presence of the building blocks of DNA in the cells. The DNA will join together by the order of the viral RNA which acts as the blue print for the new DNA. We can think of the attachments of one nucleotide to another as a string of pearls. Each pearl (nucleotide) has a hook to attach to a pre-existing pearl on the necklace and a second hook at its opposite pole to receive the pearl. The difference is that there are four kinds of pearls, and the order in which they join together is predetermined by the order found in the template RNA. This order will determine the function of each of the viral genes and whether the virus will survive even this early stage. Once the virus enters the cell it takes on a function similar to that of a Trojan horse. It switches on and begins to replicate. A virus is a small capsule made of membranes and proteins. The capsule contains one or more strands of DNA or RNA (long molecules that contain the software program for making a copy of the virus). Viruses are "life forms" which are neither alive or dead. Viruses may seem alive when they multiply, but in another sense they are obviously dead, they are only machines, but strictly mechanical. Viruses are too small to be seen. A hundred million viruses could be contained in the size of a punctuation period. This would the combined population of Great Britain and France. But it only takes one virus to infect you. A virus is a parasite. It cannot live independently. It can only make copies of itself inside a cell using the cell's material and machinery to get the job done. Viruses have a motive without a mind. Their purpose is to make copies of themselves, a job which may be executed on occasion with great speed. All living beings carry viruses in their cells. The virus being replicated inside the cell causes the cell to pop and the virus to be spilled out of the broken cell wall. Some viruses can leak through the cell wall, like a dripping water faucet.

There are two general types of retroviruses based on how they are transmitted to a host; exogenous and endogenous. Exogenous retroviruses are those that can be transmitted through the environment, for example milk that contains the BLV virus and HIV virus transmitted through blood. Endogenous retroviruses however are transmitted genetically in the germ cells (sperm and egg of animals) in the form of DNA provirus. These endogenous proviruses are ubiquitous (everywhere). They are found in every vertebra species that has been checked for them. These proviruses have a segment of them that is called the long terminal repeat (LTR) that is responsible for the movement of the genetic elements and can change from one position to another in a normal cell's DNA. So an endogenous retrovirus may have the full capacity to produce a virus. It may do so with the likelihood of eventually yielding variants that become infectious for the same animal species, or even escaping into a new species by changing itself from an endogenous to an exogenous retrovirus. This may lead to disease, particularly if the new host had not had this type of infection with this specific retrovirus in the past. Some clinical investigators and epidemiologists indicate that a retrovirus like HTLV may even promote, and perhaps directly cause, several other disorders. These include some neurological diseases, and other diseases such as rheumatoid arthritis-like disease and some muscle inflammations. [184]

## AIDS VIRUS

The AIDS virus reached epidemic proportion very quickly. The virus is relatively unstable and there can be considerable variation or mutation even in a single person infected with it. It spontaneously alters its character as it moves through populations and individuals. It can mutate during the course of even one infection. A person who dies of HIV is usually infected with multiple strains which have all arisen spontaneously throughout the body. In 1994 more than 16 million adults and one million children have been infected by the AIDS virus, a

200

virus unknown to humanity prior to 1981. Clearly the familiarity or length of time a virus has been recognized has no bearing on the amount of danger it signals. Simply because retroviruses are not generally treated with as much concern as AIDS does not void their effects from being similarly drastic.

## SUMMARY

We eliminated smallpox in the world. It will be much easier to eliminate the Bovine leukemia virus in Cows. This should be done because many of the viruses, previously thought not to cause cancer, are now known to cause cancer. These viruses can hide for years inside our cells. Epidemiologists have found this detail to make conclusive studies extremely challenging because of the difficulty of showing that a population of people having cancer today, is due to a virus that they were exposed to 10 to 20 years ago. [185]

The World Trade Organization has crippled the abilities of various countries to restrict the food which enters their markets. Society cannot guarantee the same public health inspection standards worldwide because of the greed, fraud, and deception that is prevalent in the inspection process. Therefore, there is an increased potential that diseases, or viruses, will generate large-scale, even global epidemics. We are caught in the food chain whether we like it or not. If we do not protect our food supply and try to eliminate the retroviral epidemic in cows undoubtedly we will be unprepared for the coming plague. The problems are serious and are getting worse. It is time to sound an alarm before the health dangers can multiply any further. Abundant sources of genetic variation exist for viruses to learn new tricks. Viral paths are by no means confined to where they have led in the past, or even to what we are aware occurs routinely today.

Why don't we now eradicate the bovine leukemia virus and the bovine AIDS virus from the one food that we consume more than any other, which is milk? It is up to consumers to demand by the nature of their purchases, and their support of protective legislation, that decisive measures be taken.

201

# CHAPTER 7

# SALMONELLA AND BACTERIAL INFECTIONS

## INFECTION MOVES UP TO THIRD LEADING CAUSE OF DEATH

Infectious disease deaths is on the rise in the United States in spite of historical predictions that these deaths would continue to decline. Between 1980 and 1992, the death rate from infectious diseases increased by 58%, moving from the fifth to the third leading cause of death, according to a study by the Centers for Disease Control and Prevention.[186] Overall, deaths increased by 20% for respiratory tract infections and 83% for septicemia (blood poisoning), according to the study of all U.S. death certificates filed during the 12-year period.

Microbiological food-borne disease has steadily been increasing for decades not only in the United State, but also in Europe and many other affluent countries or areas. There are now over five million cases of it per year in the US--resulting in thousands of deaths and costs of around $23 billion.

## ZOONOSIS

Most if not all of the recently emerging  infectious food-borne diseases of humans discovered in the past 50 years have been Zoonosis. In general these organisms occur in animals that look healthy but actually are carriers of disease.

Our knowledge of how these organisms react has also been evolving.  Not many years ago we thought that foods kept refrigerated (below 45 degrees F) would spoil after a period of time but that there was no significant danger of disease germ growth while at that temperature. But then we found out that Yersinia species, a significant cause of disease, including chronic rheumatoid problems and others mentioned by Dr. Douglas Archer, grows well at 40 degrees F and above. Yersinia enteocolitica is now an important pathogen in foods. Listeria species, the cause of severe disease and death especially of pregnant women and their fetuses grows well at 39 degrees F and above. Also Clostridium botulinum, type E grows above 38 degrees F, Vibrio parahaemolyticus above 43 degrees F, enterotoxigenic E. coli above 39 degrees F and Aeromonas hydrophilia above 40 degrees F. Cheese aged over 60 days recently was considered safe from living pathogens, we now know salmonella and others do survive far longer than 60 days. We also used to believe that it took hundreds of thousands if not millions of these organisms to cause disease in a healthy adult. We now know that as low as 100 organisms of some salmonella species can cause disease. As low as 100 Listeria will cause disease in about 10% of persons exposed and other infective doses are slowly being revised downward.

## SALMONELLA IN MEAT, MILK, CHEESE AND EGGS

Control and eventual elimination of salmonella from poultry products has been the goal of researchers and the poultry industry for over 25 years. Other countries have eliminated the problem but we have not, and one reason is our practice of feeding dead, disabled chickens to chickens. Salmonella is a major health problem and economic burden in the U.S. and the world. Salmonella is a bacteria that is found in manure and fecal material of infected animals. Approximately 65,347 human cases of salmonella in the U.S. in 1985, reported was quite high due to over 16,284 confirmed cases from Salmonella typhrimurium which contaminated pasteurized milk in Chicago alone.

Most people, have no idea that meats, poultry, and sea food should be considered already contaminated with one or more serious pathogens which will rub off on their hands, sinks, counter, cutting boards, knives, etc. and then contaminate the next item touched. Studies of retail meats have shown that 2-45% of all meat is positive for salmonella.

## CASES OF FOOD POISONING

How many people actually get salmonella food poisoning? (Roberts estimates 800,000 human cases plus 800 deaths of people per year in the U.S. in which the victim contracted salmonella from beef or chicken.)[187] Salmonella is still increasing and probably causing several thousand deaths per year and millions of cases of disease in the U.S. Recent studies have now identified it as the leading cause of acute bacterial gastroenteritis in the U.S. Common symptoms are diarrhea, abdominal pain, fever, excessive gas, bloating and vomiting.

A major outbreak of illness caused by Salmonella typimurium between September 17 and 30, 1984, at least 423 cases of gastrointestinal illness were investigated. One hundred and forty patients were founded to have stool cultures positive for salmonella.[188]

In June 1982 an outbreak of salmonella gastroenteritis occurred on a farm in Wyoming. All eight affected persons became severely ill 8-18 hours after they had eaten homemade ice cream. A previously healthy 13-year-old boy died 37 hours after exposure; his mother and four younger siblings were transferred to intensive care units in hospitals in adjoining states, and the remaining two adult males were hospitalized locally. This reminds us that foods from animal reservoirs, like eggs, remain in important source of salmonella. Salmonellosis can be a severe disease even in persons who are not at the extremes of age or immunocompromised.[189]

Health food fans love it, but California health officials have found that raw milk -- that has not been pasteurized to destroy germs--can make you ill or even kill you. Consumer Reports notes that the State's Department of Health Services reported that the risk of illness caused by salmonella dublin, a particularly virulent strain of salmonella bacteria, is 158 times greater among raw milk drinkers than among the general population. The number of cases in California has tripled from 1980 to 1983. Case histories taken from 99 of those people revealed that nearly half drank raw milk. One-fourth of the reported cases resulted in death. The very old, the very young, and the sick are most likely to die from salmonella dublin, which causes fever and severe diarrhea. San Francisco pediatrician Dr. John C. Bolton lead the fight against the sale of raw milk, which he calls "a habitually contaminated product." The U.S. Centers of Disease Control gives it a bad bill of health too: "There is a wealth of evidence that unpasteurized milk is associated with human disease." Consumer Reports also advises against drinking raw milk.. Since the large Chicago outbreak of salmonella in contaminated pasteurized milk, it is obvious that one can get salmonella from improperly pasteurized milk also. That the number of salmonella dublin cases in California is not larger than it is relates to the fact that the population that drinks Certified Raw Milk appears to be intermittent. Salmonellosis from raw milk is a potential hazard that merits greater appreciation by consumers, producers, and health care providers [190]

## WHY POTENTIAL FOR DISEASE?

There has been a revolution in the potential for disease from farm or sea to your table in the last 40 years. Since then, there has been a massive technological change in every stage of handling fresh meat from farm to table, except in control of pathogens (disease organisms) for which there has been a concomitant standstill or even backsliding. Animals are now fed contaminated feeds from all over the country, are raised in monstrous close-quartered numbers, are commingled in feed lots from around the country, are further commingled at slaughter plant holding pens, then are further cross-contaminated in the slaughter plants (beef, pork, chicken, etc.).

Production lines go so fast that the equipment furthers the accidental fecal contamination. Water temperature in the scald tanks is so low that it essentially kills nothing. All this is then further cross-contaminated by the cutting up, grinding up and mixing that is now common. Finally these mixed-up products are refrigerated, shipped, and received by the retail outlets, sometimes under variable temperature conditions. They then are held and sold as fresh for many days.

## BEEF

Microbiological contamination of animal carcasses during slaughtering procedures is an undesirable but apparently is a unavoidable problem in the conversion of live animals to meat for consumption. Proper dressing procedures at the abattoir can prevent a significant amount of fecal contamination, although contamination will still occur even in the best managed slaughter facilities. Much of the initial contamination of red meat carcasses comes from the hide during removal, especially when the hide is removed by mechanical means. The exposed surface of the hide and the hair accumulates dust, dirt, and fecal material during the animal's life; and this material is the primary source of bacterial contamination during slaughter. However, pathogens such as salmonellae, Campylbacter jejuni, and listeria monocytogenes can be present. There is an extreme variation in amounts of manure adhering on individual tissue surfaces. [191]

## EGGS

In the case of salmonella enteriditis (SE)--a recent strain proving difficult to combat--its effects can be fatal, especially for very young or old people. The main problem with this particular salmonella strain is that it can be transmitted through a chicken's egg, making it extremely difficult to control if equipment such as egg conveyor belts are contaminated.

The rising public health concern about SE, associated with the consumption of under cooked Grade A table eggs, is well documented. The increasing number of human SE outbreaks, especially in the northeastern and mid Atlantic states, has been viewed with concern. The total number of human cases has risen six-fold in the past ten years. Other countries, such as Great Britain, have experienced even greater levels of SE, and the World Health Organization has characterized SE as an international epidemic of grave concern.[192] In a study in Georgia, USA 50% of one day old Baby chicks were found to have salmonella contamination on hatching, before having contact with feed or the environment.[193] The National Research Council stated: "There is conclusive evidence that microorganisms pathogenic to humans (such as salmonella and Campylobacter) are present on poultry at the time of slaughter and at retail."

There were hysterical reactions in the United Kingdom following publicity on salmonella problems in the British egg industry. The British government's advice not to consume raw eggs or only eat fully cooked eggs caused an enormous decrease in table egg sales.

## FEEDING DEAD CHICKENS TO CHICKENS IS TO BLAME

Why do we have so much salmonella and other countries have little or none? Scientists believed in the 70's that the main source of the problem is animal protein in feed. If rendering is available all dead birds or hatchery wastes, like chicken manure, go into making poultry meal. It is not unusual for reprocessed poultry to be contaminated with salmonella, which means that healthy animals and birds consume infected feed from diseased dead chicken. These chickens then become a host to the diseased organisms which in turn are then passed onto humans when they consumed the eggs or chickens.[194] Thus salmonella occurs frequently in animal feed and contaminated feed has been shown to cause infection in animals and ultimately in humans.[195] [196]

Salmonella was found in the yolk sac of 9.4% of the chicks sampled with Salmonella typhimurium being the most common serotype. A high percentage of contamination has been found in slaughterhouse flies and observed that salmonella persisted from the maggot to the adult stage. While salmonella was isolated from lesser meal worms. Sixty percent of the meat and bone meal samples collected at feed mills were contaminated. Salmonella was isolated from 35% of the mash feed samples tested that were fed to chickens. [197]

## EPIDEMIC OF SALMONELLA IN CHICKENS

On February 1, 1990, the U.S. Department of Agriculture declared poultry disease caused by salmonella serotypes enteritidis (SE) to be an endemic (widespread) disease of economic and public concern. The total number of human cases has risen six-fold in the past ten years. Great Britain experienced even greater levels of SE. [198]

In the United States 6.8 million dollars were made available to the Animal and Plant Health Inspection Service to implement an SE control program.

I have been told by veterinarians visiting from other countries, speaking at scientific conventions that they are afraid to eat in our restaurants due to the large amount of salmonella in the United States. Other countries have nearly eliminated salmonella from their poultry industry. The United States has the know how to produce a clean product; it just needs to apply its knowledge. Our own Department of Agriculture admits that more than 25 percent of the chicken sold in this country has salmonella bacteria. Other estimates put the level at more than 30 percent.

## U.S. GOVERNMENT NOT TO INSPECT EGGS

Recent Epidemiologic evidence indicates that Salmonella

enteritidis (SE) infections have increased more than sixfold (1976-1986) in humans in the northeastern United States. Seventy-seven percent of the SE outbreaks reported in the Northeast were identified with Grade A shell eggs or food containing eggs. Now our government agencies have passed a law that egg shells are not to be inspected.

Between 1982 and 1987, the number of reported illnesses caused by SE in England and Wales also increased sixfold, to almost 7,000 cases. This rise in SE infections, presumably associated with contaminated shell eggs, is unlike past problems of salmonellosis associated with cracked or soiled eggs. Little is known of the Epidemiology of SE or other salmonella species in layer hens or the commercial egg production environment. It has been demonstrated that SE is translocated from the intestine to the internal organs of chicks, supporting the concept of systemic transmission of the organism. At present, Salmonella enteritidis is the cause of the systemic infection in layer hens and eggs resulting in one cause of human salmonellosis. [199]

### KILLER EGGS

Killer eggs worry health officials. Before 1979, only cracked eggs were believed to be likely carriers of the salmonella bacteria. Now it is known that it comes from the hen's ovaries and can exist in the egg's yolk, according to the Centers for Disease Control. Salmonella is the most frequently reported cause of foodborne outbreaks of gastroenteritis in the United States. Foods containing poultry or other meat, eggs, or dairy products are most often the vehicles for food-borne salmonellosis. [200]

### POULTRY INSPECTION

Just 20 companies produce 80% of American poultry, billions of tons of it annually. A high-speed production line can slaughter and gut as many as 90 chickens a minute, and the process produces much filth. Recently the industry has come under fire from the press, consumers, and Congress. Conditions in processing plants can be unsanitary and inhumane, not only for poultry but for the people who work there. The USDA is responsible for meat and poultry inspection, but in the last decade inspection has reportedly been less thorough.

The USDA seal according to industry critics, is no longer a guarantee of a clean, wholesome product. [201] The Atlanta Journal-Constitution interviewed 84 federal poultry inspectors from 37 processing plants in Georgia, Arkansas, Alabama, North Carolina and Mississippi. Included were inspectors at plants operated by the eight largest poultry companies in the United States. Among the findings: 72 of USDA inspectors at the nation's largest poultry plants said the USDA seal of approval today no longer guarantees that chicken is safe to eat.

Every week throughout the Southern U.S., millions of chickens leaking yellow pus probably from arthritic joints, stained by green feces, contaminated by harmful bacteria, or marred by lung and heart infection, cancerous tumors or skin conditions are shipped for sale to consumers, instead of being condemned and destroyed, USDA inspectors said.

1. Eighty-one inspectors said that thousands of birds contaminated or stained with feces are shipped every day instead of being condemned,

2. Seventy-five inspectors said that thousands of diseased birds pass from processing lines to stores every day.

3. Seventy inspectors said that thousands of contaminated birds are salvaged by cutting away visibly diseased meat and selling the rest—much of which is also diseased—as chicken parts.

4. Forty-seven inspectors said that maggots, especially in summer months, often infest cutting and processing machinery.

Industry executives and USDA officials told the newspaper that as long as consumers thoroughly cook poultry, there is no danger of food poisoning. Even so at least five dozen of the USDA poultry inspectors said that they were so concerned that they no longer eat chicken. It would do well to follow their example.

## DANGEROUS FOOD-BORNE PATHOGENS

America's public health is being threatened by a wide variety of food-borne illnesses. Food-borne pathogens can cause diseases such as: meningitis, arthritis, Guillan-Barre syndrome, and stillbirths. From 2% to 3% of all cases of food-borne illnesses can produce life threatening consequences. The pathogens of many food-related illnesses are never identified. Rep. Christopher Shays (R, Conn.) stated at a May hearing on the safety of the U.S. food supply that, "Many food-related illnesses are treated only symptomatically, without any identification of the offending pathogen. Even when the cause of an illness is known to be contaminated food, the necessary data is not always reported by physicians and state health authorities. As a result, national surveillance data on the prevalence and sources of food-borne pathogens is obviously inadequate."

The General Accounting Office says that between 6.5 million and 81 million Americans experience food-borne illnesses each year. Approximately 9,000 people die every year because of food-borne illnesses. A little over a decade ago 140 cases of illness were reported in Los Angeles. Thirteen of these cases were meningitis and 48 cases resulted in death. The source of these illnesses was soft cheese produced in a factory contaminated with the bacteria listeria.

National, state and local health agencies monitor foodborne illnesses. Three federal agencies the Centers for Disease Control and Prevention, the Food and Drug Administration, and the Food and Safety and Inspection Service of the U.S. Dept. of Agriculture all share responsibility for the monitoring of foodborne illnesses. They are also responsible for keeping the nation's food supply safe for all Americans.

The GAO's food and agriculture director, Robert A. Robinson has indicated that these agencies often are too slow at dealing with emerging food safety issues because of fragmented jurisdictions and responsibilities. The GAO stated in an April 1992 report that poor coordination between the FDA and USDA, and disagreement about corrective actions, hindered the federal government's efforts to control salmonella in eggs for more than five years. This alone put the American public in needless health risks because of foolish bickering and government power struggles. The GAO has recommended for years that Congress stop the "crazy quilt" structure of the federal food safety system by delegating one federal agency to be responsible for monitoring food safety. Unfortunately other members feel that interagency turf battles make it highly unlikely one agency will gain complete control and authority over food safety.

Since foods are broadly distributed throughout America, and the world for that matter, contaminated food products can reach more people in more locations. Mishandling of foods along the way to human consumption can further compound the food safety problem. The production, distribution, and preparation of food in America greatly effects the health of all Americans. All levels of government and individual health personnel must work together to ensure healthy food is marketed to all consumers.[202]

## A DREADFUL BLOW

One of the last lines of defense against many infectious diseases in humans has been dealt a dreadful blow by the Food and Drug Administration. The Commissioner of the FDA, David Kessler granted approval for the use of a new antibiotic called Sarafloxin for use with chickens raised by the broiler industry. Chicken raisers want to use this antibiotic to reduce high death losses in their flocks. They feel this new drug is necessary to keep their chickens alive. The real culprits to chicken diseases and deaths are stress to overcrowding, and unsanitary conditions on factory farms; also from feeding chickens dead chickens and chicken droppings. Sarafloxin is a fluoroquinolone, a new family of miracle drugs used by the medical profession to treat humans suffering from life-threatening illnesses. Food Animal Concerns Trust's opposition to the FDA approval of Sarafloxin use on chickens is because of scientific evidence from Europe demonstrating that the use of fluoroquinolones in farm animals results in fluoroquinolone resistant bacteria.

The Center for Disease Control has grave concerns about the approval of Sarafloxin use on chickens because fluoroquinolones are the only antimicrobial agents available for treatment of epidemic shigellosis and typhoid fever in many areas of the world. These agents according to the CDC are very important antimicrobial agents for treating a variety of serious infections in patients with serious illnesses. Resistance to fluoroquinolones has already occurred in E. coli when used in organ transplant units, and in Campylobacter jejuni, a bacterium found in most chickens sold in supermarkets. The CDC has warned that even limited use of Sarafloxin will quicken the emergence of resistance, specifically in bacteria transmitted by food. These are the foods Americans will buy, prepare and eat.

## INADEQUATE SAFEGUARDS

Food Animal Concerns Trust feels the FDA's safeguards to the use of Sarafloxin to be inadequate. They find the FDA monitoring system an inadequate safeguard against abusive drug use in animals. Once an animal drug is approved and on the market, past experience shows that it is extremely difficult for the FDA to take the drug off the market. Food Animal Concerns Trust's leaders feel there is no assurance that violators will be prosecuted since the FDA lacks the authority to assess penalties for animal drug violations. The FDA must refer violations to the U.S. Department of Justice. The Justice Department rarely acts on FDA complaints.

Chicken factory farms demand more drugs when and where ever they want them for use at their whims. The recent battle cry of the factory farm is, "Give us more drugs!" Food Animal Concerns Trust's President, Robert A. Brown says, "We want healthy farm animals that do not need all these drugs."

The factory farm industry has begun its war to increase the availability of animal drugs. The factory farm industry has: One) introduced legislation to loosen the FDA's approval process on new animal drugs. This legislation would decrease the amount of information and testing needed before a drug is approved and would permit drug companies to market drugs overseas that are not approved for U.S. use. Two) lobbying for extra-label regulations that would permit wide use of drugs for beef animals for which the drug has not been approved or even tested. Three) encouraging the U.S. government officials to lift their ban on hormone treated beef, so the U.S. cattle industry can earn more money by exporting cattle products to Europe. Four) negotiating with the FDA to eradicate the testing that feed mills now have to perform on the feed they mix with drugs.

It was a sad day when the only effective U.S. Department of Agriculture sponsored program to control salmonella enteritidis ended. The Pennsylvania Egg Quality Assurance Program closed its program in January. Salmonella has increased nationally over the past five years, but there has been a drastic reduction of 50% in Salmonella enteritidis on those farms participating in PEQAP. Al Pope, the President of the United Eggs Producers (UEP) is happy to see the PEQAP end. The UEP has made their own egg quality plan. Food Animal Concerns Trust does not believe this industry friendly board will recommend testing of flocks or eggs for salmonella.

The President of Food Animal Concerns Trust, Robert A. Brown states. "Animal diseases on farms have consequences that come directly into our homes, bringing disease and death to people too. A rise in deadly foodborne pathogens has accompanied the introduction of factory farming. In the 1980's three new bacteria emerged as serious public health problems-- campylobacter jejuni, E. coli O157.H7, and Salmonella enteritidis. During the past year new serotypes of both E. coli and salmonella have appeared. These diseases for the most part do not make the animal sick, but they cause deadly illnesses when passed onto humans.". The agriculture business uses 50% of U.S. antibiotic production to increase the growth rate of farm animals. It is alarming that from 1980 to 1992 deaths due to infectious disease has increased 58%.[203]

## STREAMLINED BEEF-INSPECTION

A book called Beyond Beef by Jeremy Rifkin,[204] exposes a new streamlined beef-inspection system (SIS) now being tested by the USDA by plants that process one fifth of America's beef. The experimental new inspection is condemned by many of the USDA's own beef inspectors. In 1985 a report by the National Academy of Sciences found that USDA inspection procedures were inadequate to protect the public from meat-related diseases. The SIS sharply reduces the federal meat inspector's role in the examination of beef carcasses destined for interstate and foreign commerce. Under the new inspection, USDA inspectors examine less than 1 percent of the carcasses (they used to examine every animal); they no longer make regular checks of the carcasses for signs of disease. They are no longer allowed to look directly at the carcass or touch it with their hands to check for signs of disease. Instead, meat must be viewed in a mirror through 15 feet of steam and fog as it whizzes by—often a useless exercise. In 1990, federal meat inspectors from around the country flooded the USDA with affidavits describing abuses throughout the new inspection system. One USDA inspector, said that "meat whose disease symptoms previously would have required it to be condemned or, at most, approved for dog food now gets the USDA seal of approval for consumers. Inspector's commented that cattle with peritonitis, a bloody, mucus-like fluid in the carcass cavity, are routinely approved. Cattle with pneumonia are approved.

The intent of SIS is to turn the responsibility for inspection over to the company and its employees. The employees take their orders and get their paychecks from the company. A federal meat inspector said that "The whole idea of meat-packing companies policing themselves is ridiculous. USDA officials respond to criticism by warning the public to make sure meat is cooked well.

For its part, the USDA has been trapped in a classic conflict of interests. It is supposed to both support and regulate the beef and poultry industries. It seems that USDA only acts if the disease causes an economic impact on the animal industry, rather than representing the consumers' interests. If the consumer declines to purchase the diseased product then USDA reacts quickly.

## ANTIBIOTICS IN FEED SAFETY

Cows and other livestock live longer when their diseases are treated with antibiotics. Antibiotic treatment of chickens, cattle and dairy cows is routine. The shelf life of milk, dairy products, eggs, poultry, and meat is extended through the antibiotics given to animals. So in addition to the five billion humans in the world that might take antibiotics, there are billions of cows, chickens, pigs, cattle, sheep, ducks, and other livestock undergoing prophylactic or treatment for disease. This causes many bacteria to be come resistant to antibiotics because over 50% of all antibiotics used in the United States are given to animals. We then eat the animal products and if we then develop pneumonia or other diseases, the antibiotic prescribed by our doctor will not help because the bacteria causing our disease has become resistant to the antibiotic. It is not sensitive to the antibiotics anymore because of resistant bacteria that developed in feeding animals antibiotics.

Soon after antibiotics came into general use in the 1940's, farmers discovered that mixing these drugs with feeds would make cattle, pigs, and chickens grow faster on a given amount of food. Antibiotic feed additives are in the hundreds of million dollar business. In 1977, the Food and Drug Administration (FDA) proposed banning the routine use of penicillin and tetracycline in animal feeds. Donald Kennedy, the FDA commissioner at that time, said that the proposal was "the first step toward FDA's ultimate goal of eliminating, to the extent possible, the non-therapeutic use in animals of any drugs needed to treat disease in man." "In our view," said Kennedy, "the benefit of using these drugs routinely as over-the-counter products in animal feeds to help animals grow faster, or in prophylactic (disease-prevention) programs, does not outweigh the potential risk posed to people."

The FDA's proposal was killed by Congressional opposition, following intense pressure from the drug and livestock industries. The industries contended that there was no firm link between the use of antibiotics in animals and the occurrence of antibiotic-resistant infections in humans. Every year since 1978, Congress has tacked a provision onto the FDA's appropriation, telling the FDA not to act on the issue until more conclusive evidence is found. Now, a new study has given additional force to the FDA's case, it indicates an apparent link between resistant bacteria in animals and disease in humans.

## SALMONELLA IN MEAT AND POULTRY

A report by the USDA stated that realistic and appropriate standards to protect public health are complex but very important. Under favorable conditions, salmonella and other disease producing bacteria multiply rapidly to levels adequate to cause human disease both in the plant and after the carcass enters the market. All possible efforts should be made to minimize contamination of meats and to remove contaminated products from the food chain. Now, and for the foreseeable future, it is not possible to ensure that all raw meat products are totally free of microbial pathogens that can cause disease in humans. Inevitably, some portion of the meat supply will be contaminated with some detectable level of one or more pathogens. [205]

USDA pamphlets portray quite well that meat makes a good growth media for disease germs and which very well defines how you should keep from contaminating it at home. You are not supposed to even touch raw poultry -- or the package it comes in -- unless you are wearing plastic or rubber gloves. And after you have prepared the poultry, you are supposed to scrub down your kitchen counter and sink with a solution of chlorine bleach. In commercial food establishments there has been drastic change in the retail work force with extremely high turnover. A less stable force means less training and knowledge about how to safely handle foods creating greater potential for contamination in restaurants resulting in the potential of food poisoning when eating out. So much of this could be eliminated if we would use the same sanitary procedures that other European countries use, such as cleaning conveyor belts, not feeding the dead chickens, other dead animals and the chicken manure back to the chickens. We can not expect to have chickens, turkeys and eggs not contaminated with salmonella when we continue to feed poultry, dead chickens, manure, and other dead infected animals. Let us stop this disgusting practice now.

## DEADLY GROUP B STREPTOCOCCUS

In the late 1970's, Strep B was the most serious life-threatening disease in Neo-Natal Units (newborn nurseries) all over the industrialized world. Of these Strep B infections 75% of all infections in babies under two months of age were fatal despite aggressive antibiotic treatment. This Strep B is the Streptococcus agalactiae that is in the udders of cows and causes Mastitis (an infection of the udder where milk is produced.).

This group B streptococci causes serious or fatal infection in newborn babies, the incidence of which has greatly increased in recent years. They may also produce a broad spectrum of diseases in predisposed adults. No clear cut demarcation has been drawn between cow and human strains. However there is overlapping of strains, infection of the bovine udder by human

219

strains may occur either in nature or experimentally and an epidemiological relationship between the consumption of raw milk and levels of Group B infection has been suggested. These observations suggest that bovine milk infected with Strep. Agalactiae (group B Strep infection) will frequently infect humans.

## LISTERIOSIS

The incidence of listeriosis appears to be increasing world wide. The deadliest foodborne outbreak ever to occur in the United States also occurred in 1985 and was due to the presence of L. Monocytogenes in a Mexican style soft cheese. One year 85 people died of listeriosis, and 18,000 became sick from eating jalisco cheese produced in Los Angeles. This because of possible use of un-pasteurized milk in cheese production. Un-pasteurized milk was added to improve the flavor of the Mexican-style cheese. This outbreak involved 142 cases. 93 of them were prenatal and 49 were adults; 48 individuals died, this was comprised of 30 fetuses and newborn infants and 28 adults.

The organism is widespread, perhaps ubiquitous (always present) in certain raw foods. Sporadic cases are linked to a few foods, notably soft cheeses, undercooked chicken and poorly reheated hot dogs. Some ready-to-eat foods (green salads, cold-smoked salmon) were not sources of infection in a case control study performed by Center for Disease Control.

Only one vegetable, the carrot, has consistently been demonstrated to be negative for the presence of this microbe and as little as 1% carrot juice added to bacteriological culture broth inhibits the reproduction of L. Monocytogenes. The factors in carrot juice responsible for this activity have not been isolate, yet they appear to be destroyed by heat in that cooked carrots lose their inhibitory effect. Carrots, however, were demonstrated to produce some substance(s) inhibitory to E. coli O157:H7 similar to that reported for L. Monocytogenes. L. Monocytogenes, C. Jejuni, and E.coli O157:H7, have a number of factors in common. All appear to have small infectious doses and all are readily destroyed by proper cooking or pasteurization.[206]

## UNDULANT FEVER-BRUCELLOSIS

Undulant fever in cows and humans is caused by Brucella abortus a bacteria found in raw milk. It causes a prolonged weakness similar to chronic fatigue syndrome and it is very difficult to treat. It has been shown that Brucella abortus survives ordinary cheese making processes and the long survival of Brucella strains in various types of cheese is well known even with the aging of the cheese. The survival of Brucella abortus in cheddar cheese aged for 6 months was reported. All the cheeses in which Brucella species was found to survive were made from raw milk, or from artificially inoculated milk. The aging of cheese is not a safeguard.

Brucella abortus in areas where it has not been eradicated, may be present in the raw milk. It survives for varying periods in different cheeses, which are made from raw milk or from artificially inoculated milk, and again, storage of the cheese is not a safeguard. Brucellosis is particularly prevalent in southern Europe, Latin America, and central Asia, which can be transmitted in unpasteurized diary foods.

An epidemiology investigation in Chicago started with a 17 year old girl who had traveled to Spain with a school group three months before the onset of symptoms. After a positive Brucella antibody test done on her blood was detected, treatment with tetracycline and streptomycin (antibiotics) was started. Food history questionnaires were completed by five of the ill students and ten unaffected students. The number of times cheese was consumed was significantly higher in patients than in controls. Before the outbreak was recognized, four of the patients had seen physicians nine times and had been confined in the school infirmary for 16 days and in hospitals for 11 days.

Large numbers of brucellosis cases have been reported in travelers to Mexico, Argentina, Peru, Italy, Greece, and Iran.

In a sampling of cheese from retail shops in one area of Iran, Brucella melitensis was isolated from 8.3% of cheese collected. It is obvious that imported cheese from other countries is very dangerous because large amounts of it have not been pasteurized and may contain disease organisms that may cause disease or even death.

## RAW MILK AND CHEESE

The following groups of pathogens can be involved in manufacturing cheese made from raw milk: TB (Mycobacterium tuberculosis), Undulant fever (Brucella species), disease producing strept (Pathogenic streptococci), staph food poisoning (Coagulase positive staphylococci), severe diarrhea that may lead to death (Enteropathogenic Escherichia coli), Salmonella, Rickettsia, Virus species, Bacillus cereus, Clostridium perfringens and Clostridium botulinum (can be fatal and cause death). [207]

## STAPH INFECTION AND CHEESE

Some coagulase positive staphylococci may survive (HTST) high temperature short time pasteurization treatment of milk. Thus the bacteria may develop in the cheese and may cause toxin to be produced which is not inactivated even with boiling or cooking, and then staphylococcal food poisoning results in the individual that ingested the cheese. Therefore cheese can cause staph food poisoning with severe vomiting and abdominal pain. Survival of staphylococci of up to 15 months has been recorded. Failure to detect staphylococci in suspect cheese, however, is no guarantee of the absence of enterotoxin. It is the enterotoxin from the staphylococci bacteria that cause the food poisoning. It is not inactivated by boiling or cooking, if the toxin had already been produced it could even be in pizza.

## BUY CHEESE LABELED MADE FROM PASTEURIZED MILK

Although improved control measures have eradicated tuberculosis in cattle in some countries, in others there is still danger of transmission of M. Tuberculosis by unpasteurized milk and cheese that may have been imported from countries still infected with the disease. The importance of enteropathogenic E. coli in adult gastro-enteritis was recognized only recently. In 1971 a large outbreak of gastro-enteritis attributed to cheese contaminated with enteropathogenic E. coli occurred in the United States.

Cheese made from raw milk and aged over 60 days was, up until recently, considered safe from living pathogens, we now know salmonella and others do survive far longer than the 60 days that cheese is aged. To illustrate: thousands of cheese-eaters contracted salmonella in 1993 after consuming cheese made from unpasteurized goats' milk in France, reported in the British Medical Journal, Jan 1996. This is a warning for us not to buy any cheese that has not been pasteurized, and avoid imported cheese.

## FOOD HANDLING

In milk that is kept cold at 40 degrees F, bacteria will not increase as rapidly as in milk held at a temperature of 50 degrees F. If milk after pasteurization contains 15,000 bacteria per ml, if held at 50 degrees, for 2 days its bacterial count may be in the millions. Milk contains bacteria such as mycoplasma, streptococcus, staphylococcus and E.coli. If you want bacterial soup let your milk become warm before you drink it. At warm temperatures bacteria population in milk doubles every 20 minutes and, before long, the milk is bacterial soup.

Then there are these products, that are now being preserved with freezing, that keep bacteria alive, lower heating temperatures, using less salts, scientists have just shown that Listeria is easily killed by salt after exposure to sublethal heat or acidification, thus there is a potential for increased survival as salt levels decrease, less acid, less sugar, less nitrites, under-cooked in microwaves, being cooked rare, or not be cooked at all. The problem begins, at least in a small way, on the farm. It proceeds to be compounded and heightened with each step leading to the ultimate consumer who indeed can make it worse. Now there are proposals to retail more refrigerated meats that have been only partially cooked along with the rare duckbreast salad, sushi, and steak tartar. A short shelf life is a consumer's protection and as shelf lives are extended so are dangers. Add to this the unknowns of the newly packaged ethnic and foreign foods being imported, that in most cases have poor inspection, and standards. Finally add the potential for genetically engineered foods to further complicate the future picture with lowered acid in tomatoes, etc., etc. Making the above more of a threat is the actual decreased education of the American consumer as to what dangers lurk in the shadows of their meat cases. To this day most people cook pork well because they have been educated about trichinosis.

## CAMPYLOBACTER

Campylobacter is common in raw milk and is found frequently in milk tanks at dairy farms. It is a common cause of mastitis, which is a infection of the udder of the cow. Since it can cause serious human disease it is a public health problem if milk is not pasteurized properly or is contaminated with raw milk.

Campylobacter (old Vibrio jejuni) was first isolated in 1909. Their significance to human disease was thought to be nil until the 1970s. A Dutch study in 1990 showed that the use of the expensive fluoroquinolone-type antibiotics (like Cipro) in chickens led to emergence of strains of the bacteria Campylobacter jejuni, and Campylobacter coli, that were resistant to the drugs in people because of the resistant bacteria in chickens and eggs.

Campylobacteriosis must now be regarded as the chief sudden cause of Guillain-Barre syndrome where humans become paralyzed, said Dr. Charles F. Bolton of the University of Western Ontario, in an editorial in the New England Journal of Medicine in November 1995. [208] [209] The patients that developed the Guillain-Barre syndrome or became severely disabled were more likely to have suffered a Campylobacter jejuni infection. People develop arm and leg weakness and occasional paralysis. This is scary because Campylobacter is a common cause of mastitis in cows and is found very frequently in milk tanks at dairies. Even though we feel it can be killed by pasteurization, the human error is involved in pasteurization of milk and raw milk may contaminate the pasteurized milk with campylobacter. None of us want the risk of being paralyzed.

One of the most frequent causes of mastitis in cows is with the infection of the bacteria Campylobacter jejuni. Mastitis or infection of the udder of the cow is the most costly disease-management complex facing the dairy industry today. Its greatest impact is in the area of lost production, followed by drug cost, increased cull rate, vet costs, and so forth. In 1976 a nationwide survey estimated that the annual loss in the United States was in excess of 1.3 billion dollars. Approximately 50 per cent of all dairy cows are afflicted with some degree of mastitis at least once per lactation.

Campylobacter was not considered a human pathogen until after 1971. Recent studies have now identified it as the leading cause of acute bacterial gastroenteritis in the U.S. Relatively small numbers (about 500 organisms) are required to cause enteritis (severe diarrhea) in man. Commonly found in healthy animal intestines, 38-56% in chickens, and 34-92% in turkeys.

Campylobacter jejuni is now considered the most frequent cause of bacterial diarrhea in the United States. The most common source outbreaks of Campylobacteriosis involve the ingestion of contaminated water or milk, although epidemiological studies implicate poultry as the vehicle of infection in the majority of cases in the U.S.

CDC data in 23 outbreaks of Campylobacter showed the

median attack rate to be 41% of those who consumed the food. The median incubation periods ranged from 66 to 120 hours after eating the infected food and the illness lasted 3-7 days. Common symptoms are diarrhea, abdominal pain, fever, excessive gas, bloating and vomiting. Though raw milk has been a major cause in the U.S. in out breaks, poultry, eggs and beef are implicated and are probably the major cause of out-breaks involving 1-3 people. A recent study by Stern showed that the presence of campylobacter jejuni and/or campylobacter coli in retail meats ranged from a low of 3.6% in ground beef to a high of 29.7% in broiler chickens. The King County Study showed up to 67% of the birds leaving the plant were positive and, among 1,936 retail meat and poultry products, an overall average 17.5% of the food products were positive. These organisms tend not to multiply readily in food at room temperature though they can survive on chilled carcasses for months. Cooking to 140 degrees F for 10 minutes will usually kill. Surveillance is still in its infancy and reporting is not required. (Roberts' estimates for Campylobacter obtained from chicken alone are 1 million human cases plus 1000 deaths per year in the U.S.)

## SCHOOL CHILDREN VISITING DAIRIES AND DRINKING RAW MILK

On May 31, 1984, twenty-eight kindergarten children and seven adults from a private school of twenty-four students in Whitter, Calif., visited a certified raw milk bottling plant in southern California where they were given ice cream, kefir, and certified raw milk. Three to six days later, several of the group began to experience fever and gastroenteritis (vomiting and diarrhea). Ultimately, nine children and three adults became ill, and most of them were absent from school. Studies on stools from these 12 persons for routine bacterial pathogens showed nine positive and three negative for campylobacter jejuni. No one else in the school became sick.

In June 1984, 17 members of a kindergarten class on Vancouver Island, British Columbia, Canada, visited a raw milk dairy; 13 drank raw milk. Nine persons became ill an average of four days after visiting the dairy. Stools from ten persons were cultured; three yielded Campylobacter jejuni. During 1983, two outbreaks of Campylobacteriosis followed consumption of raw milk on school sponsored outings in Pennsylvania. Similar outbreaks also occurred in 1981 and 1982 in Michigan, Minnesota, and Vermont. Technology does not exist to prevent contamination of raw milk supplies by Campylobacter when it is present in the intestinal tracts of about all dairy cattle. Infection may be more common than recognized, as outbreaks often are not well documented.

## SALMONELLA IN CHICAGO

The nation's worst outbreak of food-borne salmonella poisoning was linked to poor milk processing practices and the epidemic was not curtailed early due to not having a M.D. trained in public health in charge of the Health Department. This has occurred all over the United States. It occurred in one of the most sophisticated and one of the largest milk plants in the nation. In light of these facts, do you think we should be allowing our cheddar cheese to be made from un-pasteurized milk? Thirty percent of all cheese manufactured in the United States is not pasteurized and a large amount of imported cheese is not pasteurized.

## FDA's POSITION ON RAW MILK

In spite of these epidemics the FDA has refused to prohibit the retail sale of raw milk in individual states, stating that the consumer must have the right to have freedom of choice in foods. However, it has stopped the interstate shipment of raw milk. All the FDA can do is tell the people of the consequences. Do you think that a four-year old child has the ability to choose what food he eats, or that an eighty-five year old, partially senile person, who may pick up raw milk by mistake, in the grocery store, has the ability to know that the raw milk may cause disease? The FDA says it is up to the states to determine whether raw milk should be sold in their state. The Oregon State Health Department says the move for a ban on raw milk must start at the grassroots or at the county level. The public demands more than just responding to a crisis, they trust that the health department will be out there on top of these problems. The public does not realize that most milk and dairy products are inspected by the Department of Agriculture and that a conflict of interest occurs in those agencies responsible for food production, promotion, and public health regulation.

## MYCOPLASMA

Mycoplasma are organisms, intermediate between bacteria and viruses, that are capable of causing mastitis (infection of the udder) in cows. It is very difficult to grow, so special culture media is necessary if this organism is to be isolated. When it is detected in the milk tank, in all probability mycoplasma mastitis is in the milking herd. The dairyman is encouraged to detect this early, to prevent a mycoplasma mastitis outbreak in the milking herd. When humans get bronchitis, mycoplasma is many times the agent responsible and your doctor will prescribe an antibiotic like Erythromycin, Biaxin, or Zithromax that is effective on this organism.

A mycoplasma survey of goats with a history of mastitis, polyarthritis, and pneumonia revealed a high incidence of mycoplasma. During the early winter kidding season of 1979-1980, kid deaths in a large commercial dairy herd, evidenced by high fever, arthritis in many joints and pneumonia, exceeded 90%. In excess of 200 kids died. Cultures of the milk from parent does yielded 157 isolates of Mycoplasma from 605 goats (26%). Additional isolations were made from goats with polyarthritis, peritonitis, nervous disorders, and pneumonia; these animals represented 6 California counties and the states of Arizona and Idaho. Of particular importance was the observation that most milking does appeared healthy, and often milk samples were of normal appearance yet contained large numbers of mycoplasma. This milk of course was used for human consumption. The prevalence of mycoplasma in this study indicates that mycoplasmosis should be considered as one of the most important disease entities of goats in California. However, it is important to note that mycoplasma is widespread in dairy cows also. It is well known that mycoplasma mastitis spreads very easily from cow to cow. Introduction of a cow that is shedding mycoplasma in her milk is one very important way that Mycoplasma mastitis problems are established in a herd. Under the sponsorship of the California Milk Producers Advisory Board, a study investigated factors relating to the risk of herds having Mycoplasma mastitis. One study of this nature grew out of surveys for the presence of mastitis causing mycoplasma in bulk tank milks in California in 1977. At that time mycoplasma were found in bulk tank milk samples of about 3% of dairies in California. The research supported the routine use of bulk tank milk cultures for mycoplasma as a means of early detection of mycoplasma infection in a herd prior to serious outbreaks of mastitis.

## SUMMARY

From an article entitled "Food-borne Illnesses a Growing Threat to Public Health" in the June 10,1996 <u>American Medical News</u>: "Food borne pathogens- the bacteria, chemicals, viruses, parasites and unknown agents that can cause illness when ingested- pose a growing threat to the public health." Between 6.5 million and 81 million Americans experience food-borne illnesses each year and about 9,000 die as a result.

The prevalence of salmonella in America is a disgrace. We know what causes the problem. We know that the feeding practices, filth evident in the commercial meat process, lack of pasteurization and refrigeration result in infection. Is preserving traditional backward standards worth more than the thousands of lives lost in the Chicago disaster? Is the exotic taste of unpasteurized cheese worth more than the taste of a healthy life? Are the shortcuts of the poultry industry in using contaminated chickens to feed commercial chickens worth more than the personal safety of every consumer?

We have an infectious disease problem in the food animals in this country. What has allowed all this to happen? Government and public health agencies have not been placing as much emphasis on food protection. Funds were not allocated for research and enforcement. Equally important, if not most, the bureaucratic responsibilities for foods at city-county-state, federal and international levels have become so intertwined with meshed responsibilities among different agencies that no one is in charge. The result of this tangling is that even though we have known about the growing problem with salmonella since the 1950's, after each big outbreak that gets publicity the "committee effect" ensues. There is an investigation, the facts are usually obtained, and then everyone sits around self-flagellating but does nothing, due to individual interests, or fear of stepping on territorial turf. We need one agency responsible for food inspection representing the consumer and not the agriculture industry. We must insist in a clean product from healthy animals that has been produced and stored carefully, pasteurized and cooked adequately.

# CHAPTER EIGHT

# BOVINE GROWTH HORMONE

Recently, man has made milk, the most nearly perfect food, into the most nearly imperfect food. Four drug companies spent over a billion dollars developing Bovine growth hormone (rBGH). Lobbying in congress allowed rBGH to be given to cows. No long term case control studies were conducted on babies or children who drink milk to see what effects it might have on their growth or their hormone development.

The USDA seems unable or unwilling to stop the use of hormones in milk or the contamination of meat by literally hundreds of chemical additives and pollutants. In an article in the Sacramento News and Review, Feb. 15, 1996, entitled "Mystery Meat", Howard Lyman, a former Beef rancher, was asked about the government being trusted to guarantee the safety of meat. He stated, "If you're going to rely on the government to protect you from what's in the food you eat you're going to end up in Forest Lawn." Forest Lawn is a cemetery!

The increasing use of the milk stimulating hormone bovine somatotropin (rBGH) in the United States is seen as a major challenge to the European Unions policy on the use of the hormones. In February 1994 a drug company began selling the genetically engineered rBGH after a 90-day moratorium imposed by the US Congress. Activists responded by dumping milk in the streets, defacing dairy billboards, initiating a boycott and asking local school districts not to give children milk from dairies that used the hormone. At that time many dairy cooperatives and milk processors opposed the drug and told grocers that they would not be supplying milk from cows treated with the hormone. As many as 80 percent of milk processors in California, the highest-producing dairy state, are said to have either required or asked their supplies not to use the treatment. The FDA said that the hormone is safe for cows and that its presence in milk will not hurt humans. But the FDA required companies producing rBGH to print labels about hormones alerting farmers that rBGH would increase udder infections and other health problems in cows that will require medication.[210] Soon dairies and milk plants were sued for placing labels and refusing to sell rBGH milk. This had the effect of scaring others from labeling the milk rBGH free. With a lot of advertising by the drug company, the result is that 70% of the cows in the United States are receiving hormone injections. While it remains banned in the European Community, rBGH has been officially approved in the US and has been marketed here since the end of 1993.

In the U.S.A. a significant proportion of the milk being sold on the home market is already likely to have been produced by cows treated with the rBGH. Since so much milk produced by the help of rBGH is consumed in the U.S.A., the EU is having greater difficulty in blocking the import of dairy products on health grounds than it did in banning the import of hormone-treated beef from the U.S.

German milk processors have placed themselves solidly against rBGH by introducing a 12 month ban on rBGH. Secretary of State at the Ministry of Food, Wolfgang Groble, wants a seven year moratorium placed on use of the drug in milk production. Buenos Aires is siding with the Europeans and against the United States in a trade dispute under consideration by the World Trade Organization. Washington is challenging a European Union ban on the import of American beef because it's produced by feeding cattle artificial growth hormones, a practice outlawed in Europe. In what is by now a familiar refrain, U.S. officials claim the ban on U.S. beef imports was imposed simply to protect European beef producers. Germany strongly denies this and says it is banned because of health reasons.

At present, the FDA warns that rBGH-free labeling would at best be misleading, if not down right false, and it confirms the safety of dairy products originating from cows that have received supplemental rBGH shots. As pooling is a common practice, almost all milk deliveries will be, as some see it, tainted with rBGH.

I do not believe that dairy products made from animals treated with rBGH are safe, but as so often with these things it may be decades before we really know. The hormone will make cows work harder which will probably mean that they will be under greater stress, have more mastitis and won't live as long.

I am somewhat alarmed by the drug company's latest moves. The company has invested millions in this project and has certainly had to wait a very long time for the go-ahead. But to start slapping wrists- as it has recently in the U.S. - on dairy companies who harmlessly advertise that their products are made from milk produced by cows not treated with rBGH is heavy-handed in the extreme. Like many legal cases it seems largely designed to intimidate people from carrying out what would seem to be a fairly normal and acceptable practice of labeling food containers with their contents. But like most intimidation, it is apparently working.

Why did we spend millions of dollars slaughtering cows to reduce milk surplus and then approve of rBGH to increase production of milk from cows? It just doesn't make sense, except in terms of greed.

The drug company sued Swiss Valley Farms and other companies who are promoting their milk as rBGH-free. The drug company is also suing a dairy processor that refuses to purchase milk from cows treated with rBGH. The drug company contends that the advertisements and promotions from Swiss Valley Farms, Davenport, Iowa, falsely imply that its dairy products are safer than those made from the milk of rBGH-treated cows. The lawsuit singles out store signs that say "Swiss Valley Farms won't knowingly accept milk from rBGH-treated cows." The drug company reportedly took similar action against Pure Milk and Ice Cream Co., in Texas.

Many Europeans countries have banned rBGH. The Farm Animal Welfare Council has called for a continuation of the European Union's moratorium on the use of bovine soma-totrophin, because when rBGH is used to induce high levels of milk production, it can have severe effects on the welfare of cows, particularly in relation to the occurrence of mastitis and other diseases.

The Farm Animal Welfare Council says that mastitis inci-dence is clearly increased when dairy cows are treated with rBGH to induce high milk yield, It adds that no adequate study has been carried out to determine whether there is a similar effect in lower producing cows, nor whether rBGH it-self or the high milk yield produced by rBGH is the causal factor. However, it says, when mastitis is increased, the wel-fare of the cow is poorer no matter what the cause. Various reports exist suggesting increased lameness and other produc-tion related diseases, impaired conception, and tender injection sites. It says that adequate studies of the effects of rBGH on a wide range of welfare indicators are needed to demonstrate clearly the extent of adverse effects, and that licensing of rBGH should not be permitted in Europe until those data are available and have been fully assessed. The hormone remains banned in Europe. The European Union should be prepared to risk a trade row with the U.S. to defend its import ban on meat treated with growth-boosting hormones, said European Union Farm Commissioner, Franz Fischler, in January, 1996.

"The European citizen wants quality beef and milk with-out additives -- produced in a quality environment," said Nuala Ahern of the Green Party. "It gives the consumer confidence to know that hormones are banned in beef production in Europe," she added in a statement.

On January 18, 1996 the European Parliament voted to keep a European Union import ban on meat treated with growth-promoting hormones, stepping up a rumbling transatlantic row not to relax the ban under pressure from the Americans. The adopted text said too little heed had been paid to the motivations behind the European Union's hormone ban, namely consumer worries, questions of animal welfare, meat quality and the effect of hormones. The parliament called for a second conference on hormone use, to follow up on one held last year and to include producers, consumers, developing country groups, farmers and animal rights activists. Meanwhile U.S. Trade Representative Mickey Kantor threatened to take the long-running dispute to the World Trade Organization (WTO) to try to force the EU to lift its eight-year old ban.

The European Parliament gave the EU's Austrian Farm Commissioner massive support by voting unanimously to keep the EU ban on hormone-treated meat. Too little attention was paid to consumer fears, animal welfare, meat quality and negative economic impact, it said.

The European Commission has estimated that beef consumption could drop by at least 20 percent, or 1.6 million tons, if the ban on illegal hormones was lifted. France, eager to cool the transatlantic dispute before it harmed the meat industry, said it was preparing technical and possibly health arguments, to support Fischler's stance. U.S. Deputy Secretary for Agriculture, Richard Rominger insisted in Berlin that U.S.-approved hormones were safe. He said he would like to give consumers a fair choice of products again, if necessary through certificates of origin.

The U.S. sold meat worth $100 million each year to Europe prior to the ban and retaliated against the trade loss by imposing sanctions on an equivalent value of EU tomato, pasta and citrus fruit exports. These sanctions against European Union products are still being enforced today. European Union nations rallied around the EU Farm Commissioner to defend a ban on hormone-treated beef that costs American ranchers millions of dollars a year.

"It has nothing to do with the United States," said French Farm Minister Philippe Vasseur. "I just don't want to eat this," he said, referring to American meat, which generally comes from cattle treated with growth hormones. But EU Farm Commissioner, Franz Fischler acknowledged the 15-nation EU was facing an uphill battle if a planned U.S. legal challenge before the 124-nation World Trade Organization materializes in the summer of 1996. Fischler stressed that the 370 million consumers in the EU would not accept a lifting of the hormone ban because of health concerns.

The United States has always claimed the EU position was motivated purely by protectionism. Some 70 percent of American cattle are treated with growth hormones. Kantor's announcement came after EU Farm Commissioner, Franz Fischler told U.S. Agriculture Secretary, Dan Glickman by phone in the spring of 1996, that he would maintain the import ban imposed eight years ago.

Consumer fears in Europe, fanned by illegal trafficking in dangerous growth boosting substances and the persistent "mad cow" disease, were such that Fischler said he could not lift the ban. The murder of a senior Belgian veterinarian early last year by the "hormone Mafia" fueled public concern. Millions of Belgians shunned eating meat for the day on Feb. 20, 1996 in sympathy for the family of a government veterinary inspector murdered a year ago for his investigation into a "hormone Mafia." Karel Van Noppen was shot in the head at point-blank range in Wechelderzande, near Antwerp, after weeks of death threats. Exactly one year later, his killers have not been caught. Belgian newspapers reported that over three million people in Flanders--Belgium's Dutch-speaking northern region-had vowed not to eat meat on Tuesday. Von Noppen's murder stunned a Belgian public that had grown used to media reports of an international "hormone Mafia" operating in the country. The ring trades illegal hormones which are injected in cattle to artificially convert fat into meat. Leaner cattle bring higher prices ensuring more profits for farmers and slaughter houses. The trade still thrives even with fines. A recent Belgian television claimed the racket extended from breeders and farmers to government inspectors.

The beef hormone dispute would be an early test for the World Trade Organization, which has stronger dispute settlement procedures than its predecessor, the General Agreement on Tariffs and Trade. Under the new rules, countries cannot block WTO rulings. After the ruling there would then be a 60 day bilateral consultation period in which to make a final bid to find a solution. After that, the United States would request that the WTO set up a dispute resolution panel. Canada, Australia, and New Zealand are among other countries which allow the use of some meat hormones but they agreed to clearly label their exports to the EU - something the United States maintains it cannot do.

Some 200 Swiss and French farmers staged a protest in Geneva against the 1994 trade treaty which they argue opened the way for allowing infections like "mad cow" disease into the human food chain. A main target of the protest called by the Brussels-based European Farmers' Coordination organization was a United States effort through the World Trade Organization to compel the European Union to relax its ban on imports of hormone treated beef. The United States says the European Union ban violates World Trade Organization open trade rules because it is not backed by scientific evidence that growth-stimulating hormones used on cattle are a health hazard for humans. Fernand Cuche a member of the farmers group said "the U.S.A. and other exporting countries associated in the complaint to the World Trade Organization should reflect on the image they are giving their products."

Breast Cancer Action, a grassroots organization of breast cancer survivors and their supporters, published in their news letter of February 1996, that the political troubles for rBGH are mounting. Because of international standards setting organization in Rome, Italy Codex Alimentarious earlier this summer rejected a U.S. proposal to declare the use of rBGH is safe, posing no significant health risk. European countries besides the EU have placed a moratorium on use of rBGH as has Canada. The drug manufacturer is aggressively working to have such moratoriums lifted, but the newly published scientific information seems certain to make the drug company's task increasingly difficult. In the U.S., consumer advocacy groups are locked in pitched battles with rBGH-using dairies.

When a cow is injected with rBGH its milk production is stimulated, but not directly. The presence of rBGH in the cow's blood stimulates production of another hormone, called Insulin-Like Growth Factor 1, or IGF-1 for short. It is IGF-1 that stimulates milk production. IGF-1 is a naturally occurring hormone-protein in both cows and humans. The IGF-1 in cows is chemically identical to the IGF in humans. IGF-1 in milk is not destroyed by pasteurization. Because IGF-1 is active in humans--causing cells to divide--any increase in IGF-1 in milk raises an obvious question: will it cause inappropriate cell division and growth causing tumors? Americans in 1992 each consumed an average of 564 pounds of cows' milk and milk products, or about 1.54 pounds per person per day. Because milk is consumed in such large quantities, an increase in a growth-promoting hormone in milk is potentially a great public health danger and concern.

In the face of this growing body of scientific evidence, how long can rBGH-using dairy corporations maintain that their milk, butter and cheese are wholesome and safe beyond doubt?[212] Recently a study suggested that milk treated with synthetic bovine growth hormone rBGH can promote cancer in humans. The U.S. Food and Drug Administration (FDA) approved rBGH in 1985 for use in boosting milk production in cows. The government claims the product is safe for humans and animals, but consumer groups and scientists have expressed concerns about its safety. The hormone may put humans at risk for breast, colon and other gastrointestinal cancers. The reason is that levels of the insulin-growth factor 1 (IGF-1), which has been linked to cancer and tumor growth, are higher than normal in rBGH-treated milk. Pasteurization increases IGH-1 concentrations in milk. [213] [214]

## HORMONES ADDED TO FEED

Have you ever heard the adage "You are what you eat"? In the early '80s there was an alarming epidemic of premature puberty among children in Puerto Rico. The symptoms in children who had eaten beef from cows treated with the bovine growth hormone were alarming to the parents and bewildering to the affected children. The symptoms were; breast development in girls 6 months to seven years old, and sometimes in young boys. Five-year-olds were growing pubic hair. Ordinarily, premature thearche, as doctors call the condition, is a rare disorder, occurring in less than one out of 1,000 children. But in recent years, doctors in Puerto Rico have reported more than 700 cases, mostly in children under two. These physicians suspect that meat and milk producers are unlawfully using estrogen and related compounds, including the federally banned carcinogen diethylstilbestrol (DES), to increase milk production and heavier beef animals.

After seeing the problem grow for several years, local health officials blamed hormone additives in milk and meat, particularly in chicken. When these foods were eliminated from children's diets, the symptoms began to reverse themselves.

Frequently disasters occur in the production of dairy products, mainly through human error. The following news report gives an example of what tragedies occur.

5/27/96 LONDON - Doctors and consumer groups accused the British government of a cover-up over evidence that leading brands of baby milk contain chemicals that could impair fertility. "Mothers will find this very frightening," said Dr. John Chisholm of the British Medical Association. They have a right to know the facts so that they can choose milk that is safe." The Consumer's Association accused the government of putting commercial interests first. Fears about falling human fertility were first raised by a Danish scientist who in 1992 discovered that sperm counts among 15,000 men in 20 countries had dropped by almost half in 50 years.

5/28/96 LONDON - Anxious British parents deluged doctors and advice groups with calls for information Tuesday as a scare over formula baby milk posed another food safety crisis for a government already struggling with mad cow disease. The government and food manufacturers refused to name the nine brands of baby milk found in newly released test results to contain tiny traces of phthalates, a chemical which could impair fertility. The industry is investigating how the phthalates, which are used to soften plastics such as PVC, found their way into the powdered milk. The baby milk furor is the latest in a series of health scares which have panicked British consumers, including salmonella in chickens and eggs and listeria in soft cheese.

Everything we add to milk takes away its value to us with the one exception of Vitamin D. Why do we have to tamper with milk? It used to be called nature's most nearly perfect food. We are now making it the most nearly imperfect food.

# CHAPTER NINE

# CROHN'S DISEASE FROM MILK

## JOHNE'S DISEASE IN COWS

Crohn's disease in humans also called inflammatory bowel disease is similar to Johne's disease in cattle. Johne's (pronounced "yo-nees") disease is caused by the bacterium Mycobacterium paratuberculosis. It infects the small intestine of ruminant animals, especially cattle, sheep and goats, and there is no effective treatment. Cattle usually are infected soon after birth, but the first symptoms of disease do not appear until two to four years of age. It is a chronic, wasting condition and usually fatal. There is no adequately sensitive test available for the individual dairyman to test his livestock. The government does not help dairymen to rid their herds of livestock with Johne's disease as it does with tuberculosis. In the advanced stages of Johne's disease cows are thin, emaciated, and may be near death.

Johne's disease is found in every country on planet Earth! For instance New Zealand reports that paratuberculosis is widespread in dairy and beef cattle, goats and sheep. Japan has reported an annual average of 212 cases of paratuberculosis over the last five years. It is believed that the entire world has been infected with Mycobacterium paratuberculosis! Johne's disease affects a large number of cud chewing animals (ruminants) on all continents. Initially the infected cows show no symptoms, but later they develop chronic diarrhea. Diseased cows also shed large quantities of bacteria into the environment posing an ecological threat to other mammals living in the same habitats. [216]

241

Johne's disease is characterized by a chronic enteritis that is caused by gastrointestinal infection. It can be carried by cows that may appear healthy, to intractable diarrhea, severe malnutrition, dehydration, and eventual death of cattle infected with Mycobacterium paratuberculosis[217]

## HEALTH AND ECONOMIC PROBLEMS FOR HUMANS

Some humans may be ill because of eating infected meats and dairy products. Diagnostic tests for paratuberculosis are also used in Crohn's disease, a chronic inflammatory disease of the intestines and bowel mimicking Johne's disease, in which isolates identified as Mycobacterium paratuberculosis have been found in human bowel specimens. [218]

Paratuberculosis is the most serious chronic bacterial disease of ruminants. It causes severe economic losses for the dairyman. At the present time there is a rising interest among veterinarians and other scientist to study M. Paratuberculosis. [219] The yearly losses due to the disease were estimated to exceed $1.5 billion in the United States alone! Moreover, since Johne's disease is one of the most widespread bacterial diseases of domestic animals, its impact on the world economy is enormous.[220]

M. paratuberculosis is characterized by incredible diarrhea and heavy fecal shedding of bacteria. As a Dairy Herd Improvement Associate or Cow Tester, I would observe cows that were ill. I was forced to dodge the diarrhea from cows when they would raise up their tails and the fecal diarrhea would shoot out eight to ten feet in the dairy barn! Dairy inspectors do not have the time or the funding to keep cows that are sick from being milked! Contaminated milk is going into tanks containing milk that will be sold for human consumption. Currently milk tanks are so large that dairy inspectors can not detect blood infected milk, because it is so diluted. In the past, when milk was stored in ten gallon cans, the blood was easily detected. The dairyman will also inject the udders of cows suffering from mastitis with antibiotics. These antibiotics can then be transferred to milk supplies being sold to the public, which may render these same antibiotics useless in the treatment of human diseases. Calves can also be infected by ingesting colostrum and milk from paratuberculous cows.

## PREVALENT IN FIFTY PERCENT OF HERDS

A random sample of Wisconsin dairy herds stratified by herd size were tested for paratuberculosis. One hundred and fifty-eight herds of cattle were tested of which, fifty percent of these herds tested positive for paratuberculosis. There were 4,990 cattle tested of which, 7.29% tested positive for paratuberculosis. These test results should alarm the milk drinking and beef eating people of the world. Calculation of true prevalence from the apparent prevalence indicated that 4.79% of cattle and 34% of the Wisconsin dairy herds tested had serologic evidence of paratuberculosis. Among the fifty-four herds classified as positive on the basis of true prevalence estimation, the mean number of cattle who tested positive was 20.3%. [221]

## ISOLATED FROM MILK

The isolation of Mycobacterium paratuberculosis from udder tissue, supramammary lymph nodes, and milk of cows with clinical signs of paratuberculosis has been reported.[222] The mechanism of the shedding of organisms into milk presumably occurs by blood or lymphatic spread. However there is evidence that udder tissue may be infected with Mycobacterium paratuberculosis . Also, the spread of Mycobacterium paratuberculosis from the bowel to other organs in the body has been reported. [223]

## HUMAN EXPOSURE IN EARLY CHILDHOOD

In his presentation, Dr. M. T. Collins, a research veterinarian with the University of Wisconsin School of Veterinary Medicine in the Department of Pathobiological Sciences, said that the highest attack rate of Crohn's disease is in people fifteen to thirty years of age. Collins stated, "Investigators interpret this information to imply that human exposure to an agent or environmental factor, or factors, in early childhood lead to the disease." Mycobacterium paratuberculosis, the causative agent of Johne's disease (a chronic enteritis in ruminants), has been suspected to be involved in Crohn's disease in humans. Diagnostic tests for paratuberculosis are also used in Crohn's disease, a chronic human ileitis mimicking Johne's disease, in which isolates identified as Mycobacterium paratuberculosis have been found.[224]    Multiple studies in various centers have isolated Mycobacterium paratuberculosis from humans using the PCR test.  The Polymerase chain reaction test is used to detect the presence of IS900 DNA sequences specific to Mycobacterium paratuberculosis genomes in biopsies and surgical resection from fifty-three children with various gastrointestinal diseases and disorders.   IS900 sequences were found in thirteen of eighteen samples from patients with Crohn's disease. These results appear to support the hypothesis that Mycobacterium paratuberculosis is involved in the pathogenesis of Crohn's disease.[225] This pathogen, Mycobacterium paratuberculosis, can be chronically shed from the milk of asymptomatic animals. Therefore, favorable conditions exist for the transmission of these dreadful diseases from animals to humans.  Children are especially susceptible to diseases caused by contaminated dairy products because of their large consumption of dairy products, such as milk and ice cream.   Who would ever have thought that a childhood favorite could be so harmful to children?

Scientific evidence suggests a Johne's human health link. Mycobacterium paratuberculosis has been isolated from tissue taken from patients with Crohn's disease and has been implicated in the etiology of this disease. [226]  Fifteen percent of patients who suffer from Crohn's disease have first degree relatives who have had the disease. Diarrhea occurs at some time in most patients.  Crohn's disease patients have some or all of these symptoms: abdominal pain, abdominal tenderness, abdominal mass, weight loss and arthritis.  Intestinal obstruction occurs in one-third of the patients who have Crohn's disease and arthritis in five percent. Intestinal obstruction is a common problem for patients with Crohn's disease. Abscesses are another problem these patients must endure. The average Crohn's patient needs surgery every seven to eight years. After four surgeries the patient usually dies. Sadly, the life span of the Crohn's diseased patient is greatly shortened.

Medical records show the incidence of Crohn's disease is rising. The prevailing opinion is that Crohn's disease is an autoimmune disease. Patients with Crohn's disease symptoms are treated with anti-inflammatory drugs. The treatment is consistent with the treatment of any autoimmune disease. Autoimmunity is a condition characterized by an immune response against the body's own tissues. Treatment is temporary and does not result in a cure. Patients have the condition for life. Collins said that Johne's disease and Crohn's disease are remarkably similar in clinical signs and intestinal pathology. As the degree of intestinal pathology progresses, it is common to surgically remove a segment of the affected bowel. The detection of IS900 DNA in the tissues of other patients with various gastrointestinal disease might reflect an environmental exposure to Mycobacterium paratuberculosis, which could be spread from infected cattle through milk or water.[227]

Crohn's disease has long been suspected of having a mycobacterial cause. Mycobacterium paratuberculosis is a known cause of chronic enteritis (disease of small bowel) in animals, including primates, but is very difficult to detect by culture. The PCR test has greatly enhanced our ability to detect Mycobacterium paratuberculosis. IS900 is a multicopy genomic DNA insertion element highly specific for M. paratuberculosis.

## ANTIBODIES IN MILK

The ELISA test is an enzyme test that can detect antibodies in milk and blood for diagnosis of Mycobacterium paratuberculosis infection in dairy cattle and milk. The ELISA test could detect antibodies in blood and milk with comparable accuracy. It is much easier to check milk than to draw blood from a cow. [228]

## PCR CAN DETECT ONE GENOME

A polymerase chain reaction (PCR) based on the five foot region of IS900 and capable of the specific detection of even a single M. paratuberculosis genome has been developed. The PCR test found a 218 base pair (bp) segment of a DNA insertion sequence, IS900, that is specific for Mycobacterium paratuberculosis. The method reliably detected fifty organism per gram of feces. It also detected 100% of all fecal specimens containing 1600 organisms per gram of feces. [229] This was applied to DNA extracts of full thickness samples of intestine removed at surgery from forty patients with Crohn's disease, twenty-three patients with ulcerative colitis, and forty control patients without inflammatory bowel disease. Stringent precautions were taken that excluded contamination artifact. M. paratuberculosis was identified in twenty-six of forty (65%) Crohn's disease, in one of twenty-three (4.3%) ulcerative colitis, and in five of forty (12.5%) control tissues. Positive samples from both the small intestine and the colon were found in patients with Crohn's disease. In the study control samples were taken from the colon only. All PCR internal control reactions were negative.

## WIDESPREAD IN HUMANS

The presence of M. paratuberculosis in a small proportion of apparently normal colonic samples is consistent with a previously unsuspected prevalence in humans. The presence of M. paratuberculosis in two thirds of Crohn's disease tissues, but in less than five percent of ulcerative colitis tissues is consistent with an etiological role for M. paratuberculosis in Crohn's disease.[230] Blood from patients with Crohn's disease revealed that Mycobacterium paratuberculosis is suggested in thirty-six percent of patients with Crohn's disease[231]

Milk and supramammary lymph node samples were obtained from asymptomatic cows infected with Mycobacterium paratuberculosis at the time of slaughter. Study findings indicated that out of eighty-one supramammary lymph node samples taken twenty-two were culture positive for Mycobacterium paratuberculosis. Of seventy-seven milk samples, nine (11.6%) were culture positive. The prevalence of supramammary lymph node or milk infection was highest with heavy fecal shedding as in diarrhea of Mycobacterium paratuberculosis and lowest with light shedding. Checking the blood of the cow was not useful for predicting the risk of suprammary lymph node or milk infection. Shedding of Mycobacterium paratuberculosis occurs in the milk of infected cows without symptoms but, apparently less frequently than previously reported for symptomatic cows. [232]

## DON'T SHOOT THE MESSENGER

Mike Collins began his message to both the Johne's Disease Committee meeting and the general session of the U.S. Animal Health Association the same way, "Don't shoot the messenger. "Dr. M.T. Collins is a research veterinarian with the University of Wisconsin School of Veterinary Medicine in the Department of Pathobiological Sciences. His specialty is Johne's disease in cattle. This past summer, he was the program chair for an international Mycobacterium paratuberculosis meeting held in England, the Fourth International Colloquium on Paratuberculosis. Mycobacterium paratuberculosis is the organism that causes Johne's disease in cattle and a host of other ruminants. As program chair, Collins had the opportunity to review the papers presented at the conference. What he reviewed and what was presented should be of concern for dairy farmers and consumers of dairy products.

## ONE MILLION PEOPLE AFFECTED

Crohn's disease in humans, also called inflammatory bowel disease, is one of two similar conditions of the intestinal tract. It is a chronic, low-grade inflammation of the terminal (end part of) ileum; the ileum is the distal (near the end) portion of the small intestines. There is no cure. About 1 million people in the United States are affected. Each year there are 25,000 new cases in the United States.

Since Crohn's disease is not reportable, it is difficult to confirm the incidence. From 20,000 to 25,000 new cases are thought to occur in the United States each year. The incidence of Crohn's disease, four to eleven  new cases per 100,000 population, is similar to most developed countries. Current records show the incidence is rising.

### PATIENTS HAVE CONDITION FOR LIFE

The treatment of the disease is consistent with the prevailing opinion that a condition characterized by an immune response against the body's own tissues. Treatment is temporary and does not result in a cure. Patients have the condition for life. As the degree of intestinal pathology progresses, it is common to remove surgically a segment of the affected bowel.

### LACKS CELL WALL

In the late 1980's investigators began reporting isolation of Mycobacterium paratuberculosis from patients with Crohn's disease. They found that the organism frequently was present in patients in a form not found in animals affected with Johne's disease. The form  called spheroplasts, lack the normal tough cell wall which is characteristic of Mycobacteria Spheroplasts which are fragile and easily destroyed by disinfectants. Collins said spheroplasts do not survive harsh chemical treatments which typically are used to process clinical specimens for isolation of mycobacteria. The failure to survive may explain the long history of failure to grow Mycobacterium paratuberculosis from specimens of Crohn's disease patients. Without a cell wall, spheroplasts cannot be stained for viewing under the microscope. Collins states that the lack of staining might explain why the bacterium has not been seen in biopsies of affected human bowel tissues.

## GENETIC PROBES

The use of genetic probes is a relatively new laboratory technique; probes can determine if a small sequence of genetic material is present in a sample. Collins said that results of the application of gene probes to tissue samples from Crohn's patients are causing some in the human medical community to reconsider whether mycobacteria, Mycobacterium paratuberculosis in particular, might not be the cause of Crohn's disease:

♦　　　Collins listed the following which supports that Mycobacterium paratuberculosis causes Crohn's disease:

♦　　　1. Isolation of Mycobacterium paratuberculosis from a patient with Crohn's disease was reported in 1984. The isolate, when orally inoculated into infant goats, caused Johne's disease.

♦　　　2. Since 1984, isolation of Mycobacterium paratuberculosis from Crohn's patients has been reported from almost every developed country in the world.

♦　　　3. In 1992, using newly developed genetic probes, researchers reported that twenty-six of forty Crohn's patients studied harbored Mycobacterium paratuberculosis in their intestinal tissues.

♦　　　4. In July 1994, Danish workers, also using genetic probes, reported evidence of the organism in fresh intestinal tissues in eleven of twenty-four (46 percent) Crohn's patients.

♦　　　5. French investigators reported 72 percent of eighteen Crohn's patients tested positive.

♦　　　6. Using a new blood test, workers in Spain, England and Italy have found that Crohn's patients have a significantly higher rate of positive results than do control patients.

Collins also states that research data not supporting the hypothesis come from laboratories that have not been able to isolate Mycobacterium paratuberculosis consistently from Crohn's patients or have failed to find differences in the frequency of antibody titers to Mycobacterium paratuberculosis, or other mycobacteria, between Crohn's patients and suitable controls.

## SURVIVES PASTEURIZATION

Collins said Mycobacterium paratuberculosis is found in the milk of an infected cow. One researcher has reported that the organism can survive pasteurization far better than other mycobacteria. In his laboratory, Collins reported that the pasteurization time required to kill one hundred percent of a strain of Mycobacterium paratuberculosis with which he works was nine minutes; normal pasteurization time is fifteen seconds.

At the ninety-ninth annual meeting of the United States Animal Health Association it was reported that pasteurization at 145 degrees F for thirty minutes (vat method) would kill Mycobacterium paratuberculosis but high temperature short time (HTST) pasteurization at 161 degrees F for about 15 seconds (most Grade A fluid milk is pasteurized by the HTST) would not kill the Mycobacterium paratuberculosis bacteria. The preliminary results of three different pasteurization studies suggest that Mycobacterium paratuberculosis organisms may survive normal pasteurization processes. However, no data exists to suggest that viable Mycobacterium paratuberculosis have been isolated from pasteurized milk in the marketplace. Reports from England indicate Mycobacterium paratuberculosis DNA to be present in marketed milk, but viable organisms were not found in that milk.[233] I believe the reason they could not isolate the live M paratuberculosis organism is because of the nearly impossible laboratory methods available today to get the bacteria to grow in the laboratory. There may only be one organism in ten gallons of milk and it would take a year to find that one organism. But to the rescue is the Polymernase Chain Reaction test that can detect the DNA of the Mycobacterium paratuberculosis bacteria. This should be enough proof to take steps immediately for an eradication program for this deadly disease producing bacteria and to change the pasteurization methods.

## PASTEURIZATION NOT EFFECTIVE

A report on scientific studies conducted at the University of Wisconsin, funded by the Wisconsin Milk Marketing Board, to evaluate the ability of Mycobacterium paratuberculosis to withstand pasteurization was presented by Dr. M. T. Collins. Human and animal strains of Mycobacterium paratuberculosis suspended in lactate buffer or raw milk, were tested at five different temperatures and a minimum of five different heat exposure times. The results were shown graphically as thermal death curves. Comparison of these thermal death curves to present pasteurization methods revealed that the bacteria were not killed by HTST (high temperature short time) method of pasteurization, which is the method most commonly used in the US today. Dr. Judy Stabel, indicated that these findings are in agreement with similar studies conducted at her laboratory. [234] A formation of National Johne's Working Group (NJWG) worked for one year and presented their recommendations to the group. A motion to support the drafted mission statement was not passed. Later another motion was passed at the meeting. The motion stated that more study was needed before any official action could be taken. I was disappointed that an eradication program for Johne's was not enacted immediately. New pasteurization temperatures should be required at once even if it meant pasteurization by the Vat method. This could easily be accomplished. As a pasteurizer I pasteurized milk by the vat method and I know it would not be that costly to convert to the vat method in milk plants in the United States. This would assure that the American public would be protected from the disease organism that causes many deaths yearly to our children and to adults. One of my friends has to go on renal dialysis because of Crohns disease. This could be prevented in the future, if we would only realize that this is a medical emergency. It needs to be corrected at once. It also would cut down on our high costs of medical care that is bankrupting our nation.

## MILK PRODUCERS SAY NO CRISIS

At the National Dairy Board, (NDB) Charles Garrison, director of industry relations, told Hoard's Dairyman that the promotion organization recognizes two facts: 1. If the Johne's-Crohn's tie is legitimate, NDB will help the industry deal with the situation.. In the meantime, the structure has been established to manage any publicity that may result. Packets with what currently is known about the two diseases have been distributed to those who might be contacted by the media. Last fall, the Dairy Board convened a panel of experts who have worked extensively with Mycobacterium paratuberculosis, the organism that causes Johne's disease. At that time, the answer to the question of whether or not there is a relationship between the human and animal condition was, "There is not enough information to say an emphatic "no". Following that meeting, the Dairy Board funded research (not yet completed) to find out if commercial pasteurization kills Mycobacterium paratuberculosis. Garrison said that, thus far, there have been only two articles in the U.S. general press about the possible relationship between Johne's disease and Crohns disease.[235]

The scientific evidence does not support the foregoing conclusions. There is an immediate Public Health Crisis. Pasteurize the milk properly to kill Mycobacterium paratuberculosis. Do not procrastinate. Protect our babies, our children. Do not hide the facts. How can we trust the government that is in charge of inspection, if something is not done immediately?

## FATAL INTESTINAL ILLNESS WITH DIARRHEA

As stated earlier Mycobacterium Paratuberculosis (Johne's disease) is a chronic disease in cud chewing animals with widespread mycobacteriosis. It involves extensive mycobacterial shedding, which accounts for the high contagiousness of the disease, and ends with a fatal enteritis. Decreases in weight, milk production, and fertility of dairy cows produce severe economic losses for the dairyman.

## RABBITS

Rabbits infected with Mycobacterium paratuberculosis of caprine origin (Goats) were treated with streptomycin and rifampicin in combination with levamisole for a period of two months. Complete elimination of Mycobacterium paratuberculosis from feces, intestines and mesenteric lymph nodes was observed. Effectiveness of rifampicin is attributed to its effect on lymphocyte, the primary cell involved in cell mediated immunity. Cattle, sheep and goats, if treated in the early stages of infection may recover from paratuberculosis.[237]

At the Fourth International Colloquium on Paratuberculosis held in Cambridge, England, in July of 1994, a food microbiologist from Ireland also reported that Mycobacterium paratuberculosis can withstand pasteurization conditions. At that meeting, British workers reported that twenty-one of 336 (6.25 %) of cartons or bottles of milk purchased from retail outlets throughout central and southern England tested positive for Mycobacterium paratuberculosis using gene probes. While genetic probes can not distinguish dead from living organisms, when coupled with other reports, it seems plausible that the pasteurized fluid milk supply could be contaminated with viable Mycobacterium paratuberculosis.

The ability of Mycobacterium paratuberculosis to survive pasteurization may not be required for it to be found in dairy products and to be still viable. Cheese products could contain the organism. Only thirty-eight percent of milk used in the manufacture of cheeses is subjected to any heat treatment. Furthermore, when milk is heated prior to production of many cheese products, the heating regime (sixty-five degrees C for fifteen to eighteen seconds)is far less rigorous than that used for pasteurization of milk for fluid consumption, and well below that necessary to kill Mycobacterium paratuberculosis. It is now thought that the ultra high temperatures used (instead of refrigeration) primarily in Europe where milk is sold with a shelf life of six months do not kill M paratuberculosis either. Dairy products may not be the only means for exposure of humans to Mycobacterium paratuberculosis, however, studies on the tissue distribution of Mycobacterium paratuberculosis in infected animals indicate that it is present in blood and many organs of the body. Thus, red meat also could contain Mycobacterium paratuberculosis. Lastly, when considering possible mechanisms for exposure of humans to Mycobacterium paratuberculosis, the dairy industry should not be the only focus of attention. Because paratuberculosis is most prevalent in dairy cattle, and because Mycobacterium paratuberculosis is known to be excreted in milk of infected cows, the dairy industry may be the first and hardest hit. Bovine paratuberculosis is sufficiently prevalent, and costly, to warrant increased effort to control the disease, for animal production and industry profitability reasons alone. [238]

## SUMMARY

In this chapter we have added two new words to your vocabulary; mycobacterium paratuberculosis. This area of medical information is just opening to the medical profession and to the public. Scientific evidence is mounting that there is a common link between the pathogens and the symptoms of Johne's disease in cattle and Crohn's disease in humans.

Mycobacterium paratuberculosis is added to the growing list of food-borne microbial pathogens of humans, control of paratuberculosis in animals used for food production must be a requirement. USAHA, and the FDA should take action. Mycobacterium paratuberculosis is the cause of Crohn's disease, and even an important complicating infection, and investigations confirm that it is present in foods of animal origin, the magnitude of the paratuberculosis problem as a food safety issue is profound.

Since pasteurization does not kill the M. Paratuberculosis bacteria and it will infect you, my advice is to boil or use dairy products only in cooking. You must make up your own mind as to the dangers in dairy products. If you make the right decision you will not have to worry about getting the life threatening Crohn's disease.

254

# CHAPTER TEN

# DEADLY E. COLI 0157:H7

The bacteria escherichia coli was named for the German doctor, Theodor Escherich, who first isolated the genus of bacteria belonging to the family enterobacteriaceae, tribe Eschericheae. This bacterium is the common inhabitant of the intestinal tract of man and other animals. Because of its difficult name, it is usually referred to as E. coli. E. coli 0157:H7 is a mutant form of this bacterium found specifically in the intestinal tract of cattle. For the remainder of this article, it is this mutant form that will be known as E. coli.

According to the United States Department of Agriculture, the muscle of cattle, which we eat as meat, is sterile. It is only after this meat comes in contact with the contents of the intestines or the feces of infected cattle does it become contaminated. But where does E. coli come from? When a cow is fed a downer cow that died of E. coli or other bacterial disease, the cow comes down with sepsis or blood poisoning. Blood goes to every muscle and organ of the body. It may be severely contaminated with E. coli depending on how sick the cow was. When this diseased animal is killed and rendered and made into pellets in some case the E. coli will survive the process and is fed to another cow, the E. coli and many other kinds of bacteria, parasites and viruses infect the cow that ate this feed. So beef is not sterile It is thought that cattle subjected to stress are more likely to have E. coli. And cattle become more stressed when they are rounded up on the farms and ranches, herded into semi-trucks, and hauled to slaughter houses.

Because of these abnormally small enclosures, these cattle

may defecate and urinate onto each other. Now their hides are covered with this filth as they are led to slaughter. In the slaughter houses, the cattle are stunned and hung from hooks on a conveyor line, where the first thing done is the removal of their hides. Occasionally these conveyor belts move in jerky motions causing swaying which may cause the contaminated hides to flap against the exposed meat of the animal carcass or that of a neighboring carcass. It takes only a very minute amount of contamination to infect the meat. Sometimes an entire animal carcass falls unto the filthy floor of the slaughter house and it is hung back on the line with insufficient or even no cleaning what-soever. And sometimes during the cutting of the carcass, the intestines of the animal are accidentally sliced and their contents explode over the expose meat.

But what about the meat inspectors, you ask? Unbelievable as it may seem, the meat inspection laws of this country were enacted in 1907 as holdovers from the 19th century. These laws only allow the government meat inspectors the opportunity to look, smell, and touch the meat. There are absolutely no provisions to do microscopic testing! And regrettably no one can see, smell, or feel the E. coli bacteria.

The most common meat to be infected with E. coli bacteria is hamburger meat. This is because normally the hamburger you buy is made from the meat of up to 100 different head of cattle. Usually it is not the finest top quality animals that are ground up as hamburger, but old non-milk producing cows.

It only takes a microscopic amount of meat from one in-fected animal to contaminate an entire batch of meat and then this large batch of meat is divided and sent to stores and restau-rants throughout a large geographic area. Through DNA testing it was determined that the Jack in the Box hamburger meat which killed six year-old Lauren Rudolph from Carlsbad, CA in December 1992, was the same Jack in the Box hamburger meat which killed people in the State of Washington as well as Las Vegas, NV in January and February 1993.

Up until the late 1970-'s no one had any idea of what was causing this strange illness now know as E. coli poisoning. In 1977 there was an outbreak which was traced to McDonald's hamburgers in Alberta, Canada. The symptoms were severe abdominal cramps, followed by bloody diarrhea. Some of the infected people came down with hemolytic uremic syndrome (HUS), which starts by shutting down a victim's kidneys and then attacking and shutting down just about every organ in the body. There is no cure for HUS, and it is very often fatal. Canadian medical researchers suspected that it might be the reconstituted onions used on the hamburgers. But Dr. Mohammed Karmali eventually found the correlation between the hamburger meat, the E. coli, and the sickness. Today Dr. Karmali is one of the most respected E coli. authorities in the world.

Since that noted Jack in the Box outbreak in early 1993, there have been over 50 other outbreaks in this country  the USDA believes that the incidences of E. coli poisoning are increasing. Today HUS is the leading cause of kidney failure in children. For some odd reason E. coli appears to affect primarily children and senior citizens. But that was no comfort to the family of 13 year-old Eric Mueller of Oceanside, CA who died in November 1993 after a cheeseburger at a local fast food restaurant. And it was no comfort to 18 year-old Laura Day who was stricken after eating a hamburger while attending the University of Alabama shortly before Thanksgiving 1993. Laura spent 42 days in the hospital and like the Mueller family, her family spent over one-quarter million dollars for her treatment. Today Laura is again attending the University but her family is financially ruined. The medical experts have no idea what kind of long term medical problems she will continue to suffer.

What's the answer?
The best solution to the E. coli epidemic appears to be the updating of our antiquated meat inspection laws. The Chicago-based organization S.T.O.P. (Safe Tables our Priorities) has sponsored legislation which would bring meat inspections laws up-to-date.

## PATHOGEN REDUCTION

-Pathogens are bacteria which cause disease in humans. The USDA needs to:

-Set standards for pathogens in meat based on the best scientific data.

-Require meat and poultry processors to microbially test their products before they reach consumers.

-Define acceptable standards as those protecting all consumers, including children and the elderly, not just the "average" consumer.

-Set definitions for pathogens as "adulterants" under the law meaning that they are then the government's responsibility to exclude from commerce wherever they are found.

## FARM-TO-TABLE PROTECTIONS

Current regulations focus only at slaughter and processing plants. We would require protection for the consumer from farm to table and permit USDA to:

-Trace contaminated meat to its source and thus develop animal husbandry practices that minimize the presence of harmful bacteria.

-Require slaughter and processing plants to utilize processing controls to prevent meat and poultry from contamination.

-Establish an Advisory Board to the Secretary of Inspection which would include consumers as well as industry.

-Assist states in developing and monitoring microbial standards programs in retail establishment to minimize bacterial contamination and more uniformly protect the public's health.

## ENFORCEMENT

Current enforcement tools are inadequate and have led to consumers being told to control deadly bacteria at the their table. Parents of E. coli victims have been chastised for not knowing better than to feed their children that meat that isn't fully cooked. We should keep contaminated meat and poultry off supermarket shelves and away from consumers. The USDA will then have the ability to respond quickly and appropriately to public health threats by:

-Mandatory recall authority over contaminated meat and poultry products. (Unbelievably, the current system only permits voluntary recall.)

-Withdrawing Federal certification from plants that are repeat violators.

-Mandating civil fines for meat and poultry plants that violate processing controls.

-Instituting whistleblower protection for private plant employees to protect their jobs when they report processing violations.

With this unified approach, our country will start on the road to making the hamburger meat we feed our children safe to eat. It will once again allow for the exportation of our meat to countries that currently don't accept our meat because of our inspection system and their fear of contamination.

Someday we will stop feeding cows to cows, but until that day we must do all we can to protect our most precious resource -- our children.

What we are including here are anecdotal reports, not scientific proof. However, as you read them it is not possible to ignore the painful human suffering caused by the E. coli 0157:H7. The following excerpts are a memorial to the victims and their parents who had the courage to speak out.


### MICHAEL NOLE

My son was born on December 1990 a healthy 9 lb. 14 oz. bundle of love. He died 25 months, 13 days later. In 12 days, USDA approved, E. coli 0157: H7 contaminated, undercooked hamburger, that was in a children's meal, purchased at a fast food restaurant, that my son consumed, rapidly led to HUS and eventually, his death.

All of the things my son went through were the most horrific things I have ever seen in my 8 years working in the medical field, and my most recent 2 years working in an Emergency

Room. My son had bouts of diarrhea, which rapidly became runny, painful and eventually bloody...and later all blood. He was admitted to Mary Bridge Children's Hospital in Tacoma, Washington. I had no idea what was soon to follow.

The bloody diarrhea continued throughout the night, every 3-5 minutes with screams of pain and terror with each one. We went through a diaper with each one because the blood burned his skin. In the morning, he was transferred to the pediatric ICU unit. Unknown to us, there were already children there with E.coli 0157:H7. Dialysis was needed and the decision was made to transport him to a children's hospital in Seattle that had the machines for this purpose. Before they transported him I had asked to rock him in my arms in a chair next to his bed. With the help of 3 nurses and his physician, they carried him over to me with all of his tubes, IV's and other monitoring devices and set him in my arms. I rocked him and sang our favorite songs together. One of our favorites was "Jesus Loves Me." To this day, I cannot bear to hear this song. This was the last time I held my baby in my arms.

After physicians noted he had red patches on his tummy, they thought something might have burst inside him. The suggestion was made to rush him into surgery to see if they could stop or identify the internal bleeding. When we were allowed to go in to see him he had an incision from his neck to his groin area. This was so difficult to see. He did not do well after this. He opened his eyes once and we were able to see the blue of his eyes and barely a twinkle. I told him he was Mommy's big boy and that I would love him forever and someday would be with him forever in heaven. My husband and I spent several hours with him before he died. The nurses gave me a lock of his golden hair to cherish. The case history of Michael Nole was given by his mother Diane Nole.

**JESSE FENDORF**

I am Sonya Fendorf from Shawnee, Kansas. My husband

and I have a five-year old son named Jesse, who was a victim of the E.coli 0157:H7 bacteria. On Friday, October 28, 1994, I received a call at work. Jesse had lost control of his bowels at school around 11:00 a.m. I thought he probably had the flu and would be better by Monday. He had diarrhea every twenty to thirty minutes throughout Friday evening. His stool began showing signs of blood. I called his doctor on the Saturday morning October 29. He suggested that Jesse's sickness could be the flu, assuring us the blood in a child's stool was not un-usual when he was experiencing the other symptoms like nausea and an upset stomach. The doctor told us to keep a close eye on Jesse for the next three hours. Instead of getting better, Jesse started to vomit and continued to have bloody-bowel move-ments every hour throughout Saturday evening. He was so ex-hausted from being in the bathroom for 48 hours that he had his head in the trash can while he sat on the toilet, sleeping. On Sunday morning, October 30,1994, I called Jesse's doctor again to report that there had been no improvement. He told us to take Jesse to Shawnee Mission Medical Center Emergency Room for dehydration treatment. I asked the doctor if Jesse could have gotten sick like the people who ate meat from the Jack in the Box restaurants. His response to me at the time was that, "The odds are one in a million." At Shawnee Mission they admitted Jesse, stating that he appeared to be lifeless and should be better in the morning after giving him fluids intravenously. On Monday, October 31, 1994, the doctors at Shawnee Mission hospital ran tests on Jesse and decided that he needed to be at Children's Mercy Hospital in the Infectious Disease Unit. It was a more serious matter than they had originally thought. From Monday, October 31 through Wednesday, November 2 Jesse was on the 3rd floor at Children's Mercy in the Infectious Dis-ease Unit. He had been exposed to Chicken Pox a week prior. On Tuesday, the doctors decided that Jesse needed to be put on dialysis. The doctors ran tests on Jesse's bowel samples. On Wednesday they confirmed the E.coli 0157:H7 bacteria.

My husband explained to Jesse that he would be having surgery later on that evening. The doctors were going to place a

Hickman in his chest, so Jesse would not have to have needles poking him, and have dialysis tubes installed so it could wash his body of the toxin that was making him so ill. His condition was, by that time, HUS, which stands for Hemolytic Uremic Syndrome. This disease causes, among other things, anemia and kidney damage to the point that urine production decreases or stops. Our family was struggling to understand what his diagnosis was and was becoming aware that other children had died of this disease he had contracted from eating tainted meat. Although we are still not positive where Jesse got sick, we do know that it was from bad meat at a fast food restaurant.

November 4, 1994, Jesse's 5th birthday, we received news that Jesse was getting worse. Fluid had built up around his lungs, which was impairing his breathing. A doctor in the ICU inserted a needle into Jesse's side to withdraw fluids. We felt helpless and were surrounded by many families of children in the ICU with the same look in their eyes that I had. I had to look away. Jesse stayed in the ICU until Sunday, November 6 when he transferred back to the Infectious Disease Unit. He had only been in his room for approximately eight hours when he got worse. Jesse had just begun to relax when all of the sudden he looked up with terror and cried, "Daddy, help me!" Jesse began to have a seizure. It was a grand mal seizure. Jesse's body became rigid and his eyes rolled backwards. The medical personnel rushed into Jesse's room and provided him with Dilantin to control the seizure and then replaced the tube in his throat.

The family was called to the conference room. The doctor informed us that the seizure was not uncommon. They did not, however, know what had caused the seizure and could not tell us whether there would be any lasting effects. Jesse was not moving. When he finally did awaken the next day, his ability to reach and touch things was gone. The doctors had Jesse in ICU to monitor his nervous system.

On Wednesday, November 16, 1994, Jesse was discharged from the hospital with the Hickman in his chest and dialyses tubes in his stomach. I do not feel that Jesse was ready to be released from the hospital. His balance was off and he was so thin that the bones in his knees stuck out. He had trouble walking or standing for the first few weeks. Jesse reminded me of the pictures I had seen of children that had been in concentration camps. He continued to vomit, as he had when this wrenching ordeal began. Jesse will be seeing a doctor once a month for the next year to check his kidney condition. This experience has drained us financially, as well as emotionally. To date, medical bills have reached $20,000. My husband and I wait to see if Jesse will be the energetic boy we knew before this devastating and unnecessary illness. We keep praying that the rest of the organs in his body will not suffer like his kidneys. And we desperately hope that the grand mal seizure which attacked his body did not leave any lasting effects.

The Health Department has still not contacted the possible sources of contaminated meat at the restaurants or the grocery stores, because they needed to find three people to be sick from the same place. Does someone have to die before something is done about this? WHAT ARE WE GOING TO DO!? I hope that the newly elected Congress will be effective and efficient, and that the new Congressional provisions will not unintentionally eliminate necessary food regulations such as food inspection. We, as American consumers, expect our food to be safe. I was dismayed to read that, just as USDA has finally taken some action to reduce E.coli contamination, the new chairman of the House Agriculture Committee, Rep. Pat Roberts, is calling on the new Secretary of Agriculture to halt the Department's E.coli sampling program, which he said was a "shotgun approach with no accurate science, which has been a disservice to the American meat industry." Apparently, Representative Roberts did not read the recent opinion from the U.S. District Court in Texas, which upheld the sampling program, calling it a "rational response to an emerging problem." Eliminating even this minimal step toward reducing the deadly E.coli bacteria would be a grave disservice to American consumers.. What happened to my Jesse, should not happen to anyone.

## STEPHANIE ROCK

March 3, 1993, a beautiful Florida day outside. Inside the pediatric intensive care unit the nightmare was only beginning. My 5 year old daughter, Stephanie, had just been diagnosed with HUS (hemolytic uremic syndrome). A term only recently familiar to me through the Seattle outbreak articles. Those letters, HUS, became an all to familiar reality. HUS was something you read about, something that happens somewhere else, and to someone else. What a fallacy!

I listened intently as the pediatrician described the kidney failure that was already in progress. He also explained why her skin and eyes were turning yellow, why her body was bruising to the touch and why she was only partially responsive. His final words; "It's going to get worse over the next few days." I had no idea what getting worse could mean, this was already similar to a chapter from a horror story. I did not have the slightest clue how bad Stephanie would really get, nor how fast.

Thinking back, if my daughter were taken away from me at that point, my last memories would have been of balancing her body and holding her head as she was screaming, crying, in a cold sweat, struggling to survive this fifth day of bloody diarrhea, this fifth day of hell. Parental instinct tells you to do something, but little can be done for this disease except watch a perfectly healthy child deteriorate. This must be a nightmare, why won't somebody please wake me up? Finally on day nine I began to see my daughter slowly emerging from this lifeless body. Stephanie recuperated at home for several months. Nearly three years later she still experiences medical complications such as kidney and pancreas problems. I have no idea where all of this will take us. We deal with each medical problem one by one and one day at a time.

In the many months since Stephanie's illness I have come to know many parents whose children have suffered this terrible disease. As parents, we stand by and watch our children's bodies become invaded by the mechanics of modern medicine. These children are literally attacked internally by this pathogen. Parents are tortured hour by hour. Why are we experiencing this stance at the bedside of America's children, watching them die or nearly die, for no reason except industry greed. The key word here is profit. Children are suffering, some dying and our meat industry is being allowed to carry on "business as usual." Governmental action has been slow. What was promised after Seattle is still not in place, 3 years later. The case history of Stephanie Rock was given by her mother Bonnie Rock.

## ERIC MUELLER

My son paid the ultimate price for eating one of his favorite foods. Ironically this tragedy occurred in the U. S: a country rapidly approaching the 21st century, considered by many to be a world leader. However, our meat inspection laws are holdovers from the 19th century. Can you imagine if the FAA still utilized the same aviation regulations from the age of the Wright brothers with today's jet travel? Consumers wouldn't stand for it! Neither can consumers safely stand for our government's current meat inspection standards.

Death by E.coli and hemolytic uremic syndrome is a very painful and torturous death. As a parent, I stood by and helplessly watched my only son experience incredible agony before he lost consciousness and died. Immediately before slipping into unconsciousness, Eric screamed, "Get my dad!" Those were the last words he ever said. I couldn't do anything for him. I am haunted daily by this incredible, totally senseless tragedy.

The day Eric came down with bloody diarrhea, I rushed him to our clinic where he was diagnosed with appendicitis. He was immediately admitted to our local hospital where an appendectomy was performed. His appendix was totally normal. Baffled, the doctors ordered culture tests that then erroneously detected amebiasis. With this diagnosis Eric was prescribed the powerful drug, Flagyl, and two days after his appendectomy was sent

265

home. This was Friday night, and throughout the weekend, rather than recovering, Eric only got sicker. Concerned, my wife called our doctor and Eric was further examined. Upon examination, Eric was immediately re-admitted to the hospital. His health was steadily declining, and his kidneys were beginning to fail. As I was to learn later, this is the first sign of hemolytic uremic syndrome, also know as HUS.

The doctors at our local hospital were baffled for some time as to what was happening with Eric. In desperation we called in Eric's pediatrician who had known him all his life. He knew things weren't going right, and that the drug Flagyl wasn't doing anything for him. After two days he ordered Eric's transfer to Children's Hospital in San Diego. The first evening in P.I.C.U., the chief of pediatrics and another doctors talked with me at the foot of Eric's bed. They were certain he had HUS but could not find any confirmed case of amebiasis causing HUS. I would later learn from Eric's medical records that the initial amebiasis culture was never duplicated on any subsequent tests. I would also learn that unless the latest state-of-the-art tests for E.coli, called polymerase chain reaction (or PCR) tests, were administered, the percentages of false-negative readings for E.coli were very high. The PCR tests check for the DNA in the toxins created by E.coli and have an accuracy approaching 100%. The reagents for these PCR tests are between only $6 and $8, yet I have not been able to find a single medical facility in the United States regularly performing these test, except for the CDC in Atlanta, which utilizes the test only if they fear a massive outbreak.

Children's Hospital continued to treat my son for amebiasis with Flagyl in increased dosages, but there was no improvement. Eric started receiving kidney dialysis. Less than 60 hours after he was admitted to the hospital he lapsed into the coma from which he would never awake. He was placed on a respirator and again operated on. This time an ileostomy was performed in addition to a brain shunt to relieve the pressure caused from brain swelling.

Soon the dreaded results of the neurological tests that had been performed on Eric were laid before my wife and me. Eric, who had been his class president, on the school's honor roll, captain of his soccer team, assistant coach of Nikki's soccer team, member of his school's surfing team, member of the school bank, and member of the city's all-star Little League baseball team, was now a vegetable. After a conference with the doctors and our family, on November 3, 1993, we decided to remove Eric's life support systems.

Eric's life was tragically and needlessly cut short. I have made it my mission to ensure that Eric did not die in vain. I never want to see another person suffer like Eric did. I never want to see another family go through the agony our family continues to go through whenever we walk past Eric's bedroom, see his photograph or hear the name Eric.

The meat industry states it may cost $250 million dollars if meat inspection laws are updated. Eric's hospital care cost $250 thousand dollars. If his care was average, and 5000 people a year die from contaminated meats, then we are spending $1.25 billion a year just to treat those who die. Add to that the cost of the other 97% of the people who survive food poisonings, and you can see that $250 million dollars is just a drop in the bucket in the overall scheme of realistic costs. I am convinced that every one of the 250 million Americans would gratefully spend an additional one dollar per year to bring the meat inspection standards ninety years up to date. If I could, I would pay the entire 250 million dollars myself, if it would bring Eric back. There are no excuses for the pain and agony caused by these outdated laws. This case history of Eric Mueller was given by his father Rainer Mueller.

### FLORENCE METZ

My name is Robert Metz and I am here today to tell you about my mother, Florence Metz, who died on March 24, 1994 at Scripps Green hospital in La Jolla, California. My mother was 88 years old when she was snatched away from her family after succumbing to the E.coli bacteria that invaded her body.

On March 7, 1994, my sister Marjorie purchased fresh ground beef from a local supermarket. That night she made well-cooked patties and served them to my mother. A few days later, Mother began having frequent bowel movements. On Saturday afternoon, March 12, she went to Marjorie's for dinner but complained that she did not feel like eating. By Sunday her diarrhea was more frequent. She remained in bed all day Monday. On Tuesday evening she failed to flush the toilet and Marjorie discovered the bloody stool.

My sister and I consulted my mother's physician. The initial diagnosis was severe colitis. When Mother failed to respond to treatment, the surgeon recommended emergency surgery to remove what he believed was "dead colon." We were warned that mother's chances of surviving the surgery were slim, and even if she did live, she would be burdened with colostomy for the rest of her life. Mother was coherent enough to hear and understand the options from the doctor and to make the decision to die, rather than live the remaining years in discomfort and be a burden to her family and others. The doctors feared she had only a few days to live.

The following day, Friday, March 18th, Mother slipped into a coma. It was late that same afternoon when the startling results from the bowel culture arrived, citing E.coli as the cause of her sickness. Mother was taken off the morphine drip, stimulated to wake up, and transferred to the critical care unit for a new course of treatment. We were told there was a 50/50 chance of saving her life. For the next five agonizing days we watched her, in her comatose state, fail to respond to the treatment. Her condition deteriorated steadily. Her kidneys stopped functioning and her body became swollen from the pulmonary edema. On Wednesday she stopped breathing until the nurses suctioned out enough fluid from her lungs to allow her to continue breathing. Her heart remained strong. Later that day,

Marjorie and I met with the doctors and we decided that there was no more hope. We transferred her to a private room where she died 24 hours later.

I am a regular person like any of you. It could be your children, your mother, father, or your grandparent next, unless effective measures are taken to eradicate this deadly bacterium. For some of us it is already too late.

## LAURA DAY

No one counted me. No one in my college town investigated to determine the source of the bacteria which almost took my life. No one in any health department noticed my case; I was not part of any counted outbreak. No one cultured me on time. No one made the proper diagnosis until I was almost dead. Because health care professionals in Alabama were not required to report E. coli a year ago, my disease did not become statistic in any health department network. No one in the meat industry gave a thought to someone my age, an eighteen year-old college student. No one recorded that, to date, my medical bills exceed $5,200,000 for one freshman at the University of Alabama.

When I contracted E.coli I was on full academic scholarship at the University of Alabama, majoring in international finance with a minor in German. Holding offices in the Women's Honor's Program and AIESEC, an international business organization, provided me with many new and exciting challenges. My life was promising and I felt invulnerable. Then something as simple as eating a hamburger changed everything.

November 12, 1993, my brother Joe, who also attends the University, and I went home for the weekend. I began having flu-like symptoms. My mom told me to take some cold medication and that I'd probably feel better by Monday. I was awake all night Sunday. Monday morning I called my brother to take me to the campus clinic to spend another night, in spite of the fact that the stool specimen taken in the office was nothing more than blood. Wednesday morning my condition had worsened. My parents were notified that I was being transferred to a local hospital, and my mother left home immediately to be with me. She expected to find me with a simple virus. She was appalled when she arrived to find much worse. Pallor of the skin, which accompanies E.coli was already evident. Vomiting, diarrhea, and severe stomach cramps occurred every few minutes. Injections of Demerol every four hours controlled the pain for only a few minutes at a time. I began having unbearable headaches -- a condition which would reappear many times throughout my illness. These headaches would sometimes last for days. Many nights my parents took turns all night massaging my temples, my neck, my shoulders and back trying to make the pain more bearable so that I could rest. Only occasional were my parents afforded the luxury of an uninterrupted nap on the small cots in my cramped hospital room.

The doctors informed my parents on November 20 that very little was known about TIP and its complications. Treatments would be tried one at a time until I responded to one of them--if I responded at all. If I were lucky and I was cured, we would never really know which medication or procedure was responsible.

My kidneys completely shut down. Later that morning, as I was being transferred to the Medical Intensive Care Unit (MICU), I stopped breathing. Fortunately, the nurses were able to revive me. My lungs had filled with fluid, and I was placed on a ventilator to help me breathe. Weeks of respiratory therapy followed.

As a last resort, my team of doctors decided to remove my spleen in an attempt to save my life. We would not have been as optimistic about this procedure had we known that three days before I arrived at University Hospital a 26 year-old female had died from complications of TIP. The splenectomy had made no difference in her case. Luckily, after the splenectomy my platelet count improved dramatically. I spent Christmas day sore, scarred, bruised, weak and losing hair, but relieved that I would be able to leave the hospital in a few days. I was one of the fortunate few TIP survivors.

I am back in school and have resumed a full academic and social schedule. However, I will be watching what this Congress does with meat inspection reform this year. America is going to be watching very carefully because this decision affects families on the most basic level of health and safety. Safe food should be given in any civilized society that I want to be a member of. It now has an opportunity to stop this kind of senseless human suffering.

### LAUREN BETH RUDOLPH

My name is Rone Rudolph, my only daughter Lauren, age 6 years, 10 months, and 10 days died in my arms, from consequences of eating a little children's cheeseburger, laced with cow fecal contamination, it is not appropriate under any circumstances that I, (or anyone else), be put in a position to serve children, cooked or not, contaminated food, cow Dung is cow Dung no matter how one cooks it . . . (or irradiates it), it does not belong in our food, with the appropriate reporting laws in place, and enforced guidelines for the processing and manufacturing of our meat and poultry and their inspection lines, our children's lives will not be at the expense of lax issues.

Seven days before Christmas, 1992, Lauren had a hamburger at a fast food restaurant in San Diego. Two days later Lauren did not feel well, complaining of a headache and an upset stomach, she came to me for a hug and reassurance. I gave her some Tylenol and held her until she slept.

Two days later, Lauren became increasingly nauseous and the day after that it turned into diarrhea. By nightfall it had advanced to bloody diarrhea and stomach cramping, so severe that we could no longer treat this as "common flu symptoms." The doctor was called and shortly thereafter Lauren was taken to the emergency room at one of our better known and respected hospitals. There, we were greeted by a few questions, endless waiting, a minimum number of perfunctory, and the overall feeling that the health care providers thought we were overreacting. They attempted to reassure us. They did not test for E. coli 0157.H7 -- we were told to just see her pediatrician when his office opened in a few hours. They would be expecting us, when she was released from the hospital, she was visibly weak and in great discomfort and had to be carried out to the car.

We spent Christmas night reading her Christmas stories, helping her open a few presents until she became too weak to do so, and watching her eat a dinner of ice chips every fifteen minutes. That evening when we got home we decided not to open our presents until we could do it as a family, so we would wait until Lauren got home. Later on that evening, I went upstairs to just sit for a few moments in Lauren's room. Nothing could have prepared me for what I had found. Lauren had left "Santa" a note. It said "DEAR SANTA, I DON'T FEEL SO GOOD. PLEASE MAKE ME WELL FOR CHRISTMAS. LOVE LAUREN."

The next morning, I walked into Lauren's room, her father standing by her bedside with tears in his eyes, she was tossing and turning, her condition declining rapidly. . . Lauren had been crying out to her father "I'm going to die. I know I'm going to die!" I took her hand quickly and told her "she was going to be okay. We would not let anything happen to her." An hour and a half later, Lauren had a massive heart attack at age six. All I could do was to stand there and watch the cardiac unit trying to revive her. Lauren had three heart attacks all together. All her main organs were failing one by one and she had signs of little to no brain activity. Lauren was on a live support system. On the morning of December 28th, 1992, as I Held Lauren and as the last breath of life went out of her body, I could feel a sense of my life's breath leave mine as well. The first time Lauren had been tested for E.coli 0157:H7, was at her autopsy.

So many survivors of this evil illness face tremendous life-long complication. Kidney and pancreatic transplants; the threat of AIDS from transfusions; infertility, learning disabilities, diabetes, lung damage, one survivor no longer has a lining around his heart. He is a teenager. Another faces of future needing "round the clock medical care. And she is only nine. And yet still another faced five surgeries in one years time to repair damage to her colon and intestinal area, an incredibly invasive procedure, she is 18. Ask her if this is what she envisioned her junior and senior year in High school to hold for her? I think not!

I testified before a senate sub-committee on foodborne illness. At that time, I shared many concerns, one of these concerns, was the possibility of an outbreak of E.coli 0157:H7 caused from food served at hot lunch program in one of our elementary schools, in November of 1994, this was no longer a scenario. This became a reality in New Mexico when 20 children in an elementary school were hospitalized with E.coli. They had eaten Sticks or Beef on a Stick". The hospitalized children were very sick. This time they were very lucky. No one died.

We should not be naive enough to count on "Luck" to solve this problem Escherichia coli or E.coli 0157:H7 as it is known to most of us, only through awareness, education and needed change, in areas of processing and manufacturing, as well as plant inspections of our meat and poultry industry can we effectively begin to make a difference. This needs to be coupled with each state's reporting law. Because with reportability there is traceability, and with that comes accountability. With these issues in place, there also comes preventability. Doesn't it stand to reason if you can't cure something so insidious, the least one could do would be to "prevent" it? It sickens me to think that Lauren's death could have been preventable if these issues had been in place but this unfortunately, is fact.

## E. COLI MAY GIVE YOU A RAW DEAL: DEATH

What exactly is E. coli?  It's a bacteria commonly found in cattle feces which can be spread by people and animals.  According to CDC (Centers for Disease Control and Prevention) estimates up to 20,400 cases, three-quarters of all cases are directly linked to ground beef.

If you think you can only get E.coli 0157:H7 (Escherichia coli) from undercooked hamburger meat served in restaurants, think again.  The infection, which causes diarrhea (often bloody) and abdominal cramps and sometimes even acute kidney failure resulting from hemolytic uremic syndrome (HUS), has also been traced to home-prepared hamburgers.  Roast beef, unpasteurized milk, apple cider, and municipal water have also been shown to carry E. coli.  A recent article in the New York Times reported E.coli in salami making people sick, too.  Apparently, the infection can be spread from person-to-person in child day care centers and pre-school settings as well as in nursing homes and hospitals.  As many as 20,000 people are sickened each year from E. Coli the CDC estimates.  About one-third of them are hospitalized and a few hundred die, mostly children and the elderly.

CDC reported 7/13/95 that a rare strain of E. Coli made 18 people sick after they drank contaminated milk has federal health officials worried it could become as dangerous as the deadly strain from hamburgers.  Escherichia coli 0104:H21 sickened 18 people in Montana.  In Montana, CDC investigators tested equipment at the dairy plant where the pasteurized milk was produced, but could not find the source of the microbe.

As my experience as a Milk and Dairy Inspector,  nearly all milk is contaminated with manure from cows' udders that are not cleaned properly.  Filters in the pipe line filter out most of the manure, but all the milk goes through the filter that usually has some manure on it and is contaminated with e coli.  At the milk plant, employees may not be as careful as they should be and allow raw milk to contaminate pasteurized milk, in pipelines that carried raw milk and that were not cleaned correctly. Pasteurization equipment at times becomes defective and not operated correctly. For example, in the high temperature short time pasteurization equipment a metal plate is all that separates the raw milk from the pasteurized milk. As gaskets get defective around the metal plate and a pinpoint hole develops raw milk can contaminate pasteurized milk. The retail milk is spot checked with the Alkaline phosphatase test to see if the milk was properly pasteurized. Occasionally the test will be positive indicating contamination. If this happens e coli could be present in pasteurized milk.

## SUMMARY

What can you do to keep your family safe -- or at least, safer -- from the possibility of E. coli contamination? First of all, do not eat undercooked hamburger while dining out. While preparing hamburger at home, cook ground beef until the interior is no longer pink and juices run clear. Thorough cooking of beef kills E. coli. Isolate dishes and utensils that have come into contact with uncooked ground beef, so they do not contaminate other foods. Wash your hands thoroughly after handling raw meats.

It's also wise to avoid unpasteurized beverages. Presently, 18 states allow the sale of raw milk: Arizona, Arkansas, California, Connecticut, Idaho, Maine, Massachusetts, Montana, New Hampshire, New Mexico, New York, Oklahoma, Oregon, Pennsylvania, South Carolina, Texas, Utah and Washington. If someone in your family develops symptoms of E.coli, see your physician for treatment immediately. Rapid medical intervention can save lives. It can also help prevent additional infections. Remember: undercooked meat might give you more than the "runs" -- it may give you or a family member a nasty 'run-in' with death.

**Infectious disease--A Threat to Global Health and Security.**

My comments that follow are based on an editorial by Joshua Lederberg, PhD in the Journal of the American Medical Association on August 7, 1996. June 1996 the White House adopted a new national public health policy for dealing with ominous threats of emerging and reemerging infections. Chaired by Vice President Al Gore, involving at least 6 cabinet departments, and many more independent agencies a document was made into national policy, which is a notable achievement. What is lacking is a comparable endorsement from congress. Above all, we face an ever-evolving adversary: microbes a billionfold more numerous than ourselves, vested with high intrinsic mutability and replication times measured in minutes, not years.

It is unlikely this will become law because of lobbying by agriculture, beef and milk industries. This is where you can be involved by refusing to buy food that is infected. It is the only effective way to accomplish anything at the present time. Mad cow disease, Cow leukemia, Cow Aids, E. coli, Salmonella and many other microbes have learned their own tricks of jamming and simply multiplying faster than our immune system can respond. Pitted against microbial genes, we have mainly our wits. Further progress will depend very much on "doctors" and we the people recalling and embracing the historic root of that term as docents, i.e., teachers. You, the reader of this book, can influence your family, relatives, friends and neighbors. Radio talk shows reach and influence many people. Please get involved, spread the information.

## POSTLUDE

This week I began chemotherapy for multiple myeloma with mephalin and prednisone. The treatment made me so ill, and caused me so much pain, that I don't even want to describe it to my family. God has been good to give me the time, energy, and inspiration to write this book. I hope it will help save you and those you love from cancer and other disease.

# REFERENCES

[1] Hulse, Virgil; Guess What's Coming With Dinner?, Vibrant Life

[2] BVA News, Bovine Spongiform Encephalopathy, Veterinary Record, June 23, 1990, pp 626-627.

[3] Fact Sheet Bovine Spongiform Encephalopathy, USDA APHIS, July 1991

[4] William Wustenberg and Richard Marsh, Is it Safe to Feed Meat and Bone Meal? Hoard's Dairyman, pp 944. The authors are a private animal health consultant at St. Paul, Minn, and a professor of veterinary science at the University of Wisconsin-Madison, respectively.

[5] D. Matthews, Bovine Spongiform Encephalopathy, J. Roy. Soc. Health, Feb. 1991, pp 3-5.

[6] Mark M. Robinson, John R. Gorham, and James W. Glosser, Bovine Spongiform Encephalopathy, Proceedings Ninety-Fourth Annual Meeting of the United States Animal Health Association, pp 209-213.

[7] Lyle D. Miller, DVM, PhD, Department of Veterinary Pathology, Iowa State University, Ames, IA. Proceedings of the United States Animal Health Association, Oct. 16, 1988. pp 413-415.

[8] Dawson, S., Ministry of Agriculture, Fisheries and Food, Central Veterinary Laboratory, New Haw, Welbridge, Surrey KT, UK. Bulletin of the IDF 257/1991 pp 26-28.

[9] P. Brown, P.P. Liberski, A. Wolff, and D.C. Gajdusek, Resistance of Scrapie Infectivity to Steam Autoclaving after Formaldehyde Fixation and Limited Survival after Ashing at 360°C: Pratical and Theoretical Impolications. The Journal of Infectious Diseases, 1990. pp 161, 467-472.

[10] Lyle D. Miller, DVM, PhD, Department of Veterinary Pathology, Iowa State University, Ames, IA. Proceedings of the United States Animal Health Association, Oct. 16, 1988. pp 413-415.

[11] William J. Hadlow, DVM. An Overview of Scrapie in the United States, JAMA, vol. 196, no. 10, May 15, 1990. pp 1676

[12] Foote, Warren C., Approaches to Controlling Scrapie in the United States, Proceeding Ninety-second annual meeting of the United States Animal Health Association. pp 402-411.

[13] The Economist, The British Disease, April 5, 1996. p 27.

[14] Horgan, Karin, Vegetarian Times, July 1992. p 11.

[15] The New York Times, October 8, 1991.

[16] Public Health, What can Consumers do? Vegetarian Times, July 1996, pp 16-18.

[17] Brown, P., Preece, M.A., Will, R. G., Friendly Fire in Medicine, The Lancet, vol. 340, July 4, 1992. pp 24-2G.

[18] Fact Sheet Bovine Spongiform Encephalopathy, USDA APHIS, July 1991.

[19] The Washington Post, June 26, 1990.

[20] P R Watch, A Decade of Denial, First quarter 196 p 7.

[21] Are Beef By-products Risky? Vegetarian Times July 1996, pp16-18.

[22] Marsh, R.F., Bessen, R.A., Transmissible Spongiform Encephalopathies: Impact on Animal and Human Health. (Epidemiologic and Experimental Studies on Transmissible Mink Encephalopathy) Darger Verlag, Developments in Biological Standardization (Fred Brown, Ed.), Heidelberg, June 23-24, 1992.

[23] Marsh, R.F., Bessen, R.A., Lehmann, S., Hartsough, G.R., Epidemiological and Experimental Studies on a New Incident of Transmissible Mink Encephalopathy, Journal of General Virology, 1991. pp 72, 589-594.

[24] Agscene, no. 102, Spring, 1991. BSE Experts Give Up Beef.

[25] McCullough, M.E. Total Mixed Rations and Supercows, Hoard's Dairyman 1991 pp 27.

[26] Nicholas Shoon. The Independent, May 14, 1990, Monday, Home News Page. p 3. Type of Mad Cow Disease May Exist in US Cattle

[27] Crisis over BSE, Agscen. no. 100, Sept./Oct. 1990.

[28] Boller, F., Lopez, O.L., Moosey, J., Diagnosis of Dementia: Neurology. 1989. pp 39, 76-79.

[29] The New York Times, October 8, 1991.

[30] Agscen, no. 105, Winter, 1991.

[31] William J. Hadlow, DVM, An Overview of Scrapie in the United States, JAMA, vol. 196, no. 10, May 15, 1990. pp 1676.

[32] Sterling, Bruce. Sacred Cow, Omni, 1994.

[33] PR WATCH, Apocalypse Cow: U.S. Denials Deepend Mad Cow Danger, vol. 3, no. 1, First Quarter, 1996.

[34] JAMA, May 1, 1996, vol. 275, no. 17. pp 1305. From the Centers for Disease Control and Prevention, Leads from the Morbidity and Mortality Weekly Report, Atlanta, Ga.

[35] Food and Drug Administration, Compliance Policy Guide 7126.24 (issued Oct 1, 1980).

[36] Downer cows are cows that look healthy but drop dead prematurely for unknown reasons.

[37] Marsh, RF 1992 "transmissible mink encephalopathy, scrapie and downer cow disease: potential links." Paper presented at the third International Workshop on Bovine Spongiform Encephalopathy, Bethesda, MD, December 9-10, 1992  7 pp.

[38] Marks, W. A., Cerebral degeneration's producing dementia: Importance of neuropathologic confirmation of clinical diagnoses. Journal of Geriatrics-Psychology-Neurology, 1988 Oct/Dec; 1(4);187-98.

[39] Boller, Francis et al. "Diagnosis of dementia: clincalopathologic correlations., Neurology. 1989 Jan : 39(1): 76 9.

[40] Section 402 of the Federal Food, Drug and Cosmetic Act is found at 21 U.S.C. Section 312 (1988 & 1992 Supp.).

[41] See, Environmental Defense Fund v. United States Department of Health, Education and Welfare, 428 F.2d 1083 (U.S.C.A.D.C. 1970).

[42] Cutlip, R.C., et al. Transmission of Scrappie to Cattle, 3rd Intl. Workshop on BSE, 12/9-10/92, NIH, Bethesda, MD.

[43] Marsh, Richard F. And W. J. Hadlow. "Transmissible mink encephalopathy." Rev.Sci. Tech. Off. Int Epiz. 1992. 112, 539-550: Marsh, Richard RF. And R.A. Blessed "Epidemiologic and Experimental Studies on Transmissible Mink Encephalopathy." TSE: Impact on Animal and Human Health, Karger-Ver;ag, Developments in Biological Standardization (Fred Brown, Ed.), Heidelberg, June 23-24m 1992.

[44] "CVM Recommends Restricting Use of Rendered Adult Sheep." Food Chemical News, March 12, 1993, p.4.

[45] "Is it safe to feed meat and bone meal?" William Wustenberg and Richard Marsh, Hoard's Dairyman, 1990.

[46] "Resistant to Scrapie Infectivity to Steam Autoclaving After Formaldehyde Fixation and Limited Survival After Ashing at 360 degrees Centigrade: Practical and Theoretical Implications, "Journal of Infectious Diseases, Vol. 161, pp 467-472 (1990.

[47] JAVMA, "Scrapie: minor disease by Paul Zuziak. P. 449.

[48] Collinge, John and Mark s. Palmer. "Prion diseases." Current Opinion in Genetics and Development 1992, 2:448-454.

[49] Walton, T.E. 1992 Report/memo on the scrapie/bovine spongiform encephalopathy, Consultants Group Meeting, June 22, 1992, Ames, Iowa. 4pp.

[50] Osborne, Dr. Carl, Memorandum to DAP#91396, Subject: Bovine Spongiform Encephalopathy. (FDA's) CVM Options for Control and Prevention, July 3, 1991.

[51] Gibbhs, Clarence J., et al., Recommendations of the International Roundtable Workshop on Bovine Spongiform Encephalopathy, JAVMA, Vol. 196, No. 10, May 15. 1990.

[52] Asher, David M., "Recommendations concerning the risk of bovine spongiform encephalopathy in the United States," Proceedings of an international Roundtable on Bovien Spongiform Encephalopathy, JAVMA, Vol. 196, No. 10, May 15, 1990

[53] John, R. E. "National renderers association feed safety assurance efforts," in a symposium, "Feed quality assurance, a system-wide approach," p. 67, 1990.

[54] Hope, J. Et al., "Fibrils From Brains of Cows With New Cattle Disease Contain Scrapie-Associated Protein." Nature, 336:390, 1988.

[55] Kimberlin, R. H., "Transmissible Encephalopathies in Animals," Canadian Journal of Veterinary Research, 54:30-37, 1990.

[56] Taylor, D.M."Inactivation of BSE agent," in "Symposium on Virological Aspects of the Safety of Biological Products," 1990.

[57] USDA, "Bovine Spongiform Encephalopathy Surveillance in the United States." 1993.

[58] McCaskey, P. C., "Spongiform Encephalopathy in Other Species," Toxicology Forum, 185-195, 1991.

[59] Taylor, D.M., "Inactivation of BSE Agent." In "Symposium on Virological Aspects of the Safety of Biological Products." 1990.

[60] Brown, P., P.P. Liberski, A. Wolff, and DC Gajdusek, "Resistance of Scrapie Infectivity ot Steam Autoclaving After Formaldehyde Fixation and Limited Survival After Ashing at 360 de-

# REFERENCES

grees C: Practical and Theoretical Implications," Journal of Infectious Diseases, 161: 467-472, 1989.

[61] Prusiner, S. B. Et al., "Immunologic and Molecular Biologic Studies of Prion Proteins in Bovine Spongiform Encephalopathy," Journal of Infectious Diseases, 167:602-613, 1993.

[62] Stahl, N. And S. B. Prusiner, "Prions and Prion Proteins, " FASEB Journal, 5:2799-2807, 1991.

[63] Kimkberlin, R.H., "Bovine Spongiform Encephalopathy," Scientific and Technical Review, 11(2):347-390, 1992.

[64] Detweiler, L.A., "Scrapie," Revue Scientifique et Technique, Office Internationale Epizootics, 11(2):491-537, 1992.

[65] Hadlow, W.J., R.C. Kennedy, and R. E. Race, "Natural Infection of Suffolk Sheep With Scrapie Virus," Journal of Infectious Diseases, 146:657, 1982.

[66] Lang, J., "Scrapie Progress Report," 1(1):1-4, March 15, 1993.

[67] Kimberlin, R. H., "Bovine Spongiform Encephalopathy." Scientific and Technical Review, 11(2):347-390, 1992.

[68] USDA, APHIS, "Quantitative Risk Assessment of BSE in United States," 1991.

[69] Bisplinghoff, F.D., National Renderers Association letter to Animal Protein Producers, 1989.

[70] Killer Beef, Bleifuss, Joel, "In These Times, May 9, 1993.

[71] Bleifuss, Joel  A New Plague?, In These Times May 17, 1993, p12-13.

[72] News and Reports, Control of BSE: MAFF tightens up on feed production. The Veterinary Record, July 29, 1995 p 107

[73] Wells, GAH, Dawson M, Haskins SAC, et al. Infectivity in the ileum of cattle challenged orally with bovine spongform encephalopathy. Vet Rec 1994; 135: 40-41.

[74] Patterson, W.J., Dealler, S., Bovine Spongiform Encephalopathy and the Public Health, Journal of Public Health Medicine, Vol.17, No. 3, 1995 pp. 261-268

[75] Wilesmith JW, Wells GAH, Cranwell MP, Ryan JMB. Bovine spongiform encephalopathy; epidemiological studies. VET REC 1988: 123: 638-644

[76] DeLamar Gibbons, Their Secrets, Why Navaho Indians never get Cancer, The Academy of Health, P.O. Box 497, Lava Hot Springs, Id 83246 pp 61-63.

[77] H.M. McClure, M.E. Keeling, R. P. Custer, et al. Erythroleukemia in two infant Chimpanzees fed milk from cows naturally infected with the Bovine C-Type Virus. Cancer Res. 34:2745-2757, 1974.

[78] Beware of the Cow. Lancet 2:30, 1974. Olson, C., L. D. Miller, et al. Transmission of Lymphosarcoma from cattle to sheep. J.Nat. Canc. Inst. 49:1463, 1972.

[79] Miller, J.M., M. J. Van der Maaten, The Biology of Bovine Leukemia Virus Infection in Cattle, Reprinted from Viruses in Naturally Occuring Cancers, Cold Spring Harbor Conferences on Cell Proliferation, Vol. 7, Copyright 1980 Cold Spring Harbor Laboratory, pp. 901-909.

[80] DeLamar Gibbons, Their Secrets, Why Navaho Indians never get Cancer, The Academy of Health, P.O. Box 497, Lava Hot Springs, Id 83246 pp 61-63.

[81] H.M. McClure, M.E. Keeling, R. P. Custer, et al. Erythroleukemia in two infant Chimpanzees fed milk from cows naturally infected with the Bovine C-Type Virus. Cancer Res. 34:2745-2757, 1974.

[82] Miller, J.M., M. J. Van der Maaten, The Biology of Bovine Leukemia Virus Infection in Cattle, Reprinted from Viruses in Naturally Occuring Cancers, Cold Spring Harbor Conferences on Cell Proliferation, Vol. 7, Copyright 1980 Cold Spring Harbor Laboratory, pp. 901-909.

[83] McClure, H.M., Keeling, M.E., Custer, R.P., Marshak, R.R., Abt, D.A., Ferrer, J.F. Erythroleukemia in Two Infant Chimpanzees Fed Milk From Cows Naturally Infected with The Bovine C-Type Virus. Cancer Research, Vol. 34, October 1974, pp. 2745-2757.

[84] Miller, J.M., Van Der Maaten, M.J.  The Biology of Bovine Leukemia Virus Infection in Cattle, Reprinted From Viruses in Naturally Occuring Cancers, Cold Spring Harbor Conferences on Cell Proliferation, Vol. 7, Copyright 1980 Cold Spring Harbor Laboratory, pp. 901-909.

[85] Beware of the Cow. Lancet 2:30, 1974. Olson, C., L. D. Miller, et al. Transmission of Lymphosarcoma from cattle to sheep. J.Nat. Canc. Inst. 49:1463, 1972.

[86] Burny, A., Bex, F., Chantrenne, H., Cleuter, Y., Dekegel, D., Ghysdael, J., Kettmann, R., Leclercq, M., Leunen, J.J., Mammerickx, M., and Portetelle, D.  Bovine Leukemia Virus Involvement in Enzootic Bovine Leukosis. Advances in Cancer Research, Vol. 28. Academic Press, Inc., 1978, pp. 251-311.

[87]Miller, J. M., Van Der Maaten, M.J. The Biology of Bovine Leukemia Virus Infection in Cattle, Reprinted From Viruses in Naturally Occurring Cancer, Cold Spring Harbor Conferences on Cell Proliferation, Vol. 7, Copyright 1980 Cold Spring Harbor Laboratory, pp. 901-909.

[88] Klintevail K; Ballagi-Pordany A; Naslund K; Bovine leukaemia virus: rapid detection of proviral DNA by nested PCR in blood and organs of experientially infected calves., Veterinary Microbiology 42 (1994) 191-204.

[89] Sherman, M.P., J. of Clinical Microbiology, Jan 1992

[90] The Journal of Health and Healing Interview with K.J. Donham 1981

[91] The Lancet, Nov 27, 1976, page 1184-1186

[92]Is bovine leukosis out of control? Hoards Dairyman, Thomas Howard, August 25, 1992, Page 571.

[93]Burny, A., Bex, F., Chantrenne, H., Cleuter, Y., Dekegel, D., Gysdael, J., Kettman, R., Leclercq, M., Leunen, J. J., Mammerickx, M. and Portetelle, D., Bovine Leukemia Virus involvement in Enzootic Bovine Leukosis. Advances in Cancer Research,Vol. 28. Academic Press, Inc., 1978, pp. 251-311.

[94]Donham, K. J., Van Der Maaten, J. J., Miller, J.M., Cruz, B.C., Rubino, M.J., Seroepidemiologic Studies on the Possible Relationships of Human and Bovine Leukemia. Journal of Nutritional Cancer Institute, Vol 59, 1977, pp. 851-853.

[95]Ferdinand, G.A.A., Langston, A., Ruppanner, R., Drlica, S., Theilen, G.H. and Behymer, D.E., Antibodies to Bovine Leukemia Virus in a Leukosis Dairy Herd and Suggestions For Control of the Infection. Canadian Journal of Comparative Medicine., Vol. 32, No. 2, 1979, pp. 173-179.

[96]Ferrer, J.F., M.D., Bovine Lymphosarcoma., The Compendium on Continuing Education For the Practicing Veterinarian, Vol. II, No. II, Nov., 1980 pp. 235-242.

[97]Olson, C., Progress for Control of Bovine Leukosis., The Bovine Practitioner, No. 14, Nov., 1979, pp. 115-120.

[98]Trainin, Z., Meirom, R., Barnes, A., Common Reactivity of Bovine and Human Sera Towards Bovine Lymphoid Tumor Cells. Comparative Leukemia Research, 1975 Bibl. Haematol., Vol. 43, 1976, pp 232-234.

[99]Van Der Maaten, M.J., Miller, J.M., (USDA Research Service, North Central Region, National Animal Disease Center, Ames, Iowa 50010), Current Assessment of Human Health Hazards Associated with Bovine Leukemia Virus, Cold Springs Harbor, 1977, pp. 1223-1234.

[100]Ferrer, J.F., M.D., Kenyon, S.J., Gupta, P., Milk of Dairy Cows Frequently Contains a Leukemogenic Virus, Science, Vol. 213, Aug. 28, 1981, pp 1014-1016.

[101]Sorensen, D. K., Clinical Manifestation of Bovine Leukosis Symposium, 1979. U. S. Department of Agriculture.

[102]Onions, D., Animal Models: Lessons From Feline and Bovine Leukaemia Virus Infections, Leukemia Research, Vol. 9, No 6, pp. 709-711, 1985.

[103] California Meat Inspection 1961, Bureau of Meat Inspection Division of Animal Ilndustry, California Dept of Agri. Sacramento, Calif.

[104]Miller, Janice, Update on Federal condemnation for Lymphosarcoma in U.S. S. Cattle, Proceedings of the U.S.A.H.A. Meeting, OCT 29, 1991

[105]Thurmond, M.C., Holmberg, C. H., Picanso, J. P., Antibodies to Bovine Leukemia Virus and Presence of Malignant Lymphoma in Slaughtered California Dairy Cattle. JNCI. VOL. 74, NO 3, march 1985, pp 711-714.

[106]Thurmond, M.C., Holmberg, C. H., Picanso, J. P., Antibodies to Bovine Leukemia Virus and Presence of Malignant Lymphoma in Slaughtered California Dairy Cattle, JNCI, Vol. 74, no. 3, pp. 710-714, March 1985

Burridge, M.J., D.N. Puhrk, and J.M. Hennemann. Prevalence of Bovine Leukemia Virus Infection in Florida. JAVMA 9:704, 1981.

[107]Alderson, M., Klein, G., Winehouse, S., Advances in Cancer Research. Vol. 31. Academic Press, N.Y., 1980, pp. 1-77.

[108] Linos, A., kyle, R.A., O'Fallon, W.M., and Kurland, L.T., Leukemia and Prior Malignant and Hematologic Diseases: A Case-Control Study., American Journal of Epidemiology Vol. 113, 1981, pp. 285-289.

[109] Fasal, E., Jackson, E.W., Flauber, N., Leukemia and Lymphoma Mortality in Farm Reside ts., American Journal of Epidemiology, Vol. 87, 1968, pp. 267-274.

[110] Milham, S., Leukemia and Multiple Myeloma in Farmers., American Journal of Epidemiology, Vol. 87, 1978, p. 267.

[111] Butmridyrt, L.F., Cancer Mortality in Iowa Farmers, 1971-1978. JNCI Vol. 66, No. 3, March 1981, pp. 461-464.

[112] Szklo, M., Are Further Epidemiologic Relationship of the Bovine Population and The Human Leukemia in Iowa. The American Journal of Epidemiology, Vol. 112, No.2, 1981, ppg. 225-231.

[113] Cancer Statistics, 1996. A Cancer Journal for Clinicians, American Cancer Society, Inc, Jan/Feb 1996 Vol 46 No.1

[114] Hehlmann, R., RNA Tumor Viruses and Human Cancer. Current topics of Microbiology and Imunology; 73:141-215, 1976

[115] Grant, C. R.. Tumor immunology, The Veterinary Cancer Medicine, Ed. Theilen, Lea and Feigiger, 1979.

[116] Pasqualini, C. D., International Symposium of Zoonosis and its possible Relation with Human Lymphomas and Leukemia's, Medicina (Buenos Aires)

[117] Ferrer, J.F., M.D., Kenyon, S.J., Gupta, P., Milk of Dairy Cows Frequently Contains a Leukemogenic Virus, Science, Vol. 213, Aug. 28, 1981, pp 1014-1016.

[118] Rubino, M. J., Donham, K.J., Inactivation of Bovine Leukemia Virus-infected Lymphocytes., American Journal Veterinary Research, Vol 45, No 8. pp 1553-1556.

[119] Roberts, D. H., Lucas, MH, Wibberley, G., Effect of Heat on Bovine Leukosis Virus-Infected Lymphocytes, British Veterinary Journal, Vol 139, 1983, pp 291-2

[120] Ferrer, J. F. Bovine Lymphosarcoma. The Compendium on Continuing Education for the Practicing Veterinarian, vol ii No ll, 235-242, 1980.

[121] Rubino, M.J. Inactivation of Bovine Leukemia Virus in Milk. Thesis, University of Iowa, December, 1980.

[122] Townsend, Leon, Milk Safety, Dairy and Food Sanitation, August, 1981.

[123] Rubino, M. J. Inactivation of Bovine Leukemia Virus in Milk. Thesis, University of Iowa, December, 1980.

[124] Peterson, M.S., Johnson, A.H., Encycylopedia of food science, The AVI Publishing Company, Westport, Connecticut, 1978, pp. 785-788.

[125] International Dairy Federation Bulletin, Viruses Pathogenic to Man in Milk and Cheese, 1980, pp. 17-20.

[126] Gross, Ludwik, The Role of Viruses in Cancer, Leukemia, and Malignant Lymphomas, Medical Times, vol 113, No. 9, September, 1985, pp 67-67.

[127] Buehring GC; Krame PM; Schultz RD; Evidence for bovine leukemia virus in mammary epithelial cells of infected cows, Laboratory Investigation Vol 71, No 3, p. 359, 1994.

[128] Brenner, J., Vet. Immunol. Immunopathol. 22:299-305, 1989

[129] Molloy JB: Dimmock CK: Eaves FW: Control of bovine leukaemia virus transmission, Veterinary Microbiology 1994 39 (3-4); 323-33.

[130]Meischke, H.R. In Vitro Transformation by Bovine Papilloma Virus, Journal of General Virology, 1979, Vol. 43, pp. 473-487.

[131]J.F. Evermann, P.L. Dorn, D.Derse, and J.L. Heeney, Interactions Between Bovine Herpesviruses and Bovine Leukosis Virus: Disease Implications. Proceedings of the 92nd annual meeting United States Animal Health Association Oct 1988, pp 103-111.

[132] Hailata N; johnson r; al-Bagdadi F, Proliferating cell nuclear antigen expression in sheep infected with bovine leukemia virus, Veterinary Immunology and Immunopathology , 44 (3-4): 211-22, Feb 1995.

[133] Buehring GC; Kramme PM; Schultz RD, Evidence for bovine leukemia virus in mammary Epithelial Cells of Infected Cows, Laboratory Investigation Vol. 71, No. 3, p. 359, 1994.

[134]Heath, Jr., C.W. The Significance of Leukemia Clusters. Hospital Practice, January 1968, pp. 64-70.

[135]Heath, Jr., CW, Human Leukemia: Genetic and Environmental Clusters, Comparative Leukemia Research, 1969 Bibl. Haemat., No. 36, R.M. Dutcher, pp. 649-653, Karger, Basel/Munchen/Paris/New York, 1970.

[136]Bartsch, D.C., Springher, F., Falk, K. H., Acute Nonlymphocytic Leukemia, An Adult Cluster, JAMA, Vol. 232, No. 13, June 30, 1975, pp. 1333-1336.

[137]Public Health Service CDC, Atlanta, EPI-770-36-2, January 8, 1979, Human Leuke-mia/Lymphoma Associated with Bovine Leukemia Virus Positive Dairy Herd, Woodbridge, Connecti-cut.

[138] Pullen, Michael M., Exension Veterinarian, The Bovine Leukemia Virus and Human Health, University of Minnesota, Informational Letter, not intended as a News Release, to County Extension Directors and Agents.

[139] Caldwell , RG, Seroepidemiologic testing in man for evidence of antibodies to feline leukemia virus and bovine leukemia virus. Symposium on comparative leukemia research, 1975. Bibl Haematol 43:238-241, 1976.

[140] Donham, KJ, Van DerMaaten, M. J, Miller, Jm, Seroepidemiologic studies on the possible relationship of human and bovine leukemia: Brief communication. J Natl Cancer Inst 59:851-852, 1977.

[141] Gilden, RV, Long, CW, Hanson, M, Characteristics of the major internal protein and RNA dependent polymeranse of bovine leukemia virus. J Gen Virol 29:305-314, 1975.

[142] Olson, C., Driscoll, D.M. Bovine Leukosis: Investigation of Risk for Man, JAVMA, Vol 173, No 11 pp 1470-1472/

[143]Blair, A., Hayes Jr., H.M. Cancer and other Causes of Death Among U.S. Veterinarians, 1966-1977. In. J. Cancer, Vol. 25, pp. 181-185, 1980.

[144]Blair, A., White, D.W., Death Certificate Study of Leukemia Among Farmers From Wis-consin, Journal of the National Cancer Institute, Vol. 66, June, 1981, pp 1027-1030.

[145]Donham, K.J., Berg, J.W., Sawin, R.S. Epidemiologic Relationship of the Bovine Popula-tion and The Human Leukemia in Iowa. The American Journal of Epidemiology, Vol. 112, No.1, 1980, pp. 80-92.

[146]Neil Pearce, Allan H. Smit, John S. Reif, Increased Risks of Soft Tissue Sarcoma, Malignant Lymphoma, and Acute Myeloid Leukemia in Abattoir Workers, American Journal of Industrial Medicine 14:63-72 (1988) pp 63-67.

[147]Olson, Carl. Progress for Control of Bovine Leukosis. The Bovine Practitioner, No. 14, November, 1979, pp. 115-120.

[148]Ferrer, Jorge F. Bovine Lymphosarcoma, Advances in Veterinary Science and Compara-tive Medicine, Vol. 24, 1980, pp 53-57, Academic Press, Inc., New York, N.Y.

[149] Burney, A. Advances in Cancer Research, 1978.

# REFERENCES

[150]Sorensen, D.K., Beal Jr., V.C. prevalence and Economics of Bovine Leukosis in The United States, Bovine Leukosis Symposium, May 22-23, 1979, sponsored by the U.S.D.A.

[151]Bovine Leukosis Symposium, May 22-23, 1979, University of Maryland, College Park, Maryland, sponsored by the U.S. Department of Agriculture, Animal and Plant Health Inspection Service, Veterinary Services and Science and Education Administration.

[152]Grant, C.K. Tumor Immunology. Veterinary Cancer Medicine, Ed. Gordon H. Thielen, D.V.M. and Bruce R. Madewell, D.V.M., M.S., Lea and Febiger, Philadelphia, 1979.

[153]Bovine Leukosis Symposium, May 22-23, 1979, University of Maryland, College Park, Maryland, sponsored by the U.S. Department of Agriculture, Animal and Plant Health Inspection Service, Veterinary Services and Science and Education Administration.

[154]Grant, C.K. Tumor Immunology. Veterinary Cancer Medicine, Ed. Gordon H. Thielen, D.V.M. and Bruce R. Madewell, D.V.M., M.S., Lea and Febiger, Philadelphia, 1979.

[155]Rubino, M.J. Inactivation of Bovine Leukemia Virus in Milk. Thesis, University of Iowa, December, 1980.

[156]International Dairy Federation Bulletin, Viruses Pathogenic to Man in Milk and Cheese, 1980, pp. 17-20.

[157] Peterson, M.S., Johnson, A.H., Encyclopedia of Food Science, The AVI Publishing Company, Westport, Connecticut, 1978, pp 785-788.

[158] Personal letter: Ferrer, Jorge F. M.D. Professors of Microbiology, Section of Viral Oncology, University of Pennsylvania, January 30, 1987

[159]Committee on Diet, Nutrition and Cancer, Diet, Nutrition and Cancer, National Academy Press, Washington, D.C., 1982.

[160]California Morbidity, Infectious Disease Section, State Department of Health Services, February 27, 1981.

[161]Peterson, M.S., Johnson, A.H., Encyclopedia of food science, The AVI Publishing Company, Westport, Connecticut, 1978, pp. 785-788.

[162]International Dairy Federation Bulletin, Viruses Pathogenic to Man in Milk and Cheese, 1980, pp. 17-20.

[163]Lloyd, J.O. Meeting Abstract. Journal of The American Veterinary Association, Vol. 171 (10):1099, 1977.

[164]Sorensen, D.K., Beal Jr., V.C. prevalence and Economics of Bovine Leukosis in The United States, Bovine Leukosis Symposium, May 22-23, 1979, sponsored by the U.S.D.A.

[165]Ferrer, Jorge F. Bovine Lymphosarcoma, Advances in Veterinary Science and Comparative Medicine, Vol. 24, 1980, pp 53-57, Academic Press, Inc., New York, N.Y.

[166] J. Clausen, R. Hoff-Jorgensen, HB. Rasmussen, Antibody reactivity against animal retroviruses in multiple sclerosis. Acta Neurol Scand 1990: 81 : 223-228

[167]A Altaner, V. Altanerova, J. Ban, O. Niwa, K. Yokoro, Human cells of neural origin are permissive for Bovine Leukemia Virus, Neoplasma, 36, 6, 1989 pp 691-695.

[168]Kuzmak, J., Moussa, A., Grundboeck-Jusko, J., Detection of the Bovine Leukaemia Virus by the Polymerase Chain Reaction, ACTA BIOCHIMICA POLONICA, Vol e8, No 1, 1991, p107-110.

[169] St.Cyr Coats K; Pruett SB: Nash JW; Bovine immunodeficiency virus: incidence of infection in Mississippi dairy cattle, Veterinary Microbiology 42 (1994) 181-189.

[170] Gonda MA; Luther DG; Fong SE; Bovine immunodeficiency virus: molecular biology and virus-host interactions. Virus Research 32(1994) 155-181.

171 M. J. Van Der Maaten, C. A. Whetstone, Bovine Lentivirus, 94th annual meeting of the US ANIMAL HEALTH ASSOCIATION. pp81-88.

[172] Hira N; Xuan S; Ochiai K; Alteration of immune responses of rabbits infected with Bovine Immunodeficiency-like Virus. Microbiol. Immunol., 38(12). 943-950. 1994.

173 Matthew a. Gonda, Michael J. Braun, Stephen G. Carter, Thomas A. Kost, Julian W. Bess Jr, Larry O. Arthur, Van Der Maaten, Characterization and molecular cloning of a bovine lentivirus related to human immunodeficiency virus. Nature Vol 330, Nov 26, 1887 pp388-391

[174] Hira N; Xuan S; Ochiai K; Alteration of immune responses of rabbits infected with Bovine Immunodeficiency-like Virus. Microbiol. Ilmmunol., 38(12). 943-950. 1994.

[175] Gonda MA; Bovine ilmmunodeficiency virus, AIDS 1992 6 (8) : 759-76 Aug

[176] Baron, T. D.,Mallet, F.,The bovine immnodeficiency-like virus (BIV) is transcriptionally active in experimentally infected calves, Archives of Virology (1995) 140: 1461-1467.

[177] Jacobs RM; Smith sHE; Gregory B; Detection of multiple retroviral infections in Cattle and Cross-reactivity of Bovine Immunodeficiency-like Virus and Human Immunodeficiency Virus Type 1 Proteins using Bovine and Human Sera in a Western Blot Assay, Canadian Journal of Veterinary Research; 1992, 56: 353-359.

178 Gonda, M.A., Luter, D. G., Fong, S. E., Bovine immjunodeficiency virus: molecular biology and virus-host interations, Virus Research, May 19943 32 pp 155-81

179 J.F. Evermann, P.L. Dorn, D.Derse, and J.L. Heeney, Interactions Between Bovine Herpesviruses and Bovine Leukosis Virus: Disease Implications. Proceedings of the 92nd annual meeting United States Animal Health Association Oct 1988, pp 103-111.

180 M.J. Van der Maaten, C.A. Whetstone, V.V. Khramtsov and J.M. Miller, Experimentally-Induced Infections with Bovine Immunodeficiency-Like Virus, A Bovine Lentivirus. 21st Congress of the IABS on Progress in Animal Retroviruses, Annecy, France, 1989, Develop. Biol. Standard., Vol. 72, pp. 91-95 (S. Karger, Basel, 1990)
M. J. Van der Maaten, C. A. Whetstone; Virology Cattle Research, USDA, Agricultural Research Service P.O. Box 70, Ames, Iowa 50010 Proceedings 94th Annual Meeting United States Animal Health Association October 6-12, 1990, pp 81-88

181 Foundation on Ecoomic Trends, Jeremy Rifkin, Petition to USDA, Center for Disease Control, and NIH on Bovine Immunodeficiency Virus. August 3, 1987; James Wyngaarden, B (NIH) and Bert Hawkins (USDA). Letter to Jeremy Rifkin, Foundation on Economic Trends, Washington, D.C., September 23, 1987. Foundation on Economic Trends, Petition to Dr. Bernadine Healy, NIH, Edward Madigan, USDA, and James Glosser, APHIS, USDA on BIV, BLV and Retroviruses of American Cattle, Washington, D.C.: Foundation on Economic Trends, May 31, 1991. Response by Dr. Bernadine Healy, NIH, July 18, 1991.

[182] St.Cyr Coats K; Pruett SB: Nash JW; Bovine immunodeficiency virus: incidence of infection in Mississippi dairy cattle, Veterinary Microbiology 42 (1994) 181-189.

[183] Johnson, E. Cancer Detection and Prevention Vol 18(1)09-30 (1994)

[184] Gallo, R Virus Hunting, A new republic book, a Division of Harper Colins Publishers p97, 15, 243.

[185] Garrett, Laurie, The Coming Plague, Farrar, Straus and Giroux New York 1994 p 233.

[186] JAMA 275:189-93, 1996.

[187]Edward L. Menning, DVM MPH, Zoonotic Meat/Poultry Food-Borne Microbiological Diseases; Their Increase and Selected Information. Proceedings of the 94 meeting of the U.S. Animal Health Association. pp 430443

[188]DaMassa, A.J., Brooks, D.L., Alder, H. E., Caprine Mycoplasmosis: Widespread infection in goats with Mycoplasma mycoides subsp mycoides(large-colony type) Am J Vet Res, Vol 44, No.2 pp 322325.

[189]Am. J. Epidemiol 119:907-12, 1984.

190[190]California Morbidity, Salmonella dublin in California, March 30, 1984, #12.

[191]James S. Dickson and Maynard E. Anderson, Control of Salmonella on Beef Tissue Surfaces in a Model System by Pre- and Post-Evisceration Washing and Sanitizing, with and Without Spray Chilling, Journal of Food Protection, Vol. 54, July 1991 pp 514-518.

[192]Dr. John Mason, Dr. Chester Gipson, Dr Thomas J. Holt, The Initiation of a Salmonella Serotype Enteritidis control program for Table Egg Poultry in the United States, Proceedings of the U.S. Animal Health Association 94th meeting, pp 317

[193]R.W.A.W. Mulder, Salmonella in poultry is a worldwide problem, Poultry--Misset Dec. 89-Jan 90

[194]H.C. Saxena, How to Utilize Dead Birds, Poultry--Misset Dec. 89-Jan 90 pp 23.

[195] Zecca, BC, The Dillon Beach Project: A five-year epidemiology study of naturally occurring salmonella infections in turkeys and their environment, Avian Diseases 1977, 21:141-159/

[196] McConnel, DG, Epidemiology of an international outbreak of Salmonella agona, 1973, Lancet 11, 1827: 490-493.

[197] F.T. Jones, R. C. Axtell, D. V. Rives, S. E. Scheideler, F. R. Tarver, Jr., R. L. Walker, and M. J. Wineland, A Survey of Salmonella Contamination in Modern Broiler Production, Journal of Food Protection, Vol. 54, July 1991, pp 502-507.

# REFERENCES

[198]Dr. John Mason, Dr. Chester Gipson, Dr Thomas J. Holt, The Initiation of a Salmonella Sero-type Enteritidis control program for Table Egg Poultry in the United States, Proceedings of the U.S. Animal Health Association 94th meeting, pp 317

[199]Harold M. Barnhart, David W. Dreesen, Robert Bastsien, and Oscar C. Pancorbo, Prevalence of Salmonella enteritidis and other Serovars in Ovaries of Layer Hens at Time of Slaughter, Journal of Food Protection Vol. 54, No. 7, Pages 488-491 (July 1991)

[200]CDC. Food borne disease outbreaks, 5 -year summary, 1983-1987. In: CDC surveillance summaries, March 1990. MMWR 1990;39(no. SS-1):15-57.

[201]University of California at Berkeley Wellness Letter Vol. 8, Issue 3, December 1991

[202] American Medical News, Kent, Christina . "Food-borne illnesses a growing threat to public health". p. 17.

[203] FACT ACTS, Food Animal Concerns Trust, P.O. Box 14599 Chicago, IL. 60614, Winter 1996, Vol. 6, No. 2.

[204]J. Rifkin, Beyond Beef, 1992 a book review by Longevity, December 1991,

[205]Farid E. Ahmed and Robert F. Kahrs, Evaluation of USDA's Streamlined inspection system for cattle: Public Health perspectives, Proceedings of the US Animal Health Association, 1990? pp 417-429.

[206] Madden, Joseph M., Concerns Regarding the Occurrence of Listeria monocytogenes, Campy-lobacter jejuni, and Escherichia coli O157:H7 in Foods Regulated by the U.S. Food and Drug Administration. Dairy, Food and Environmental Sanitation, Vol. 14, No. 5, Pages 262-267, May 1994.

[207]International Dairy Federation Bulletin, Behavior of Pathogens in Cheese June 1980, pages 1-33.

[208] The Veterinary Record, February 28, 1981 Another Zoonosis

[209] The changing concepts of Guillain-Barre syndrome, (editorial)N Engl J Med 1995 Nov. 23; 333 (21) : 1415-7.

[210] Nature :BST enters battle for consumers. vol. 387, Feb. 17, 1994 p585

[211] FAWC concern over BST, News and Reports, The Veterinary Record, July 9, 1994, p 27

[212] The BGH-Cancer connection; Breast Cancer Action Feb. 1996 The article is excerpted from Rachel Environment and Health Weekly, #454.

[213] Epstein, Samuel, International Journal of Health Services, Winter issue 1995,

[214] Vegetarian Times; BGH linked to cancer in humans March 1996, page 18

[215] Westendorf, M L; There are no Johne's disease quick fixes, Hoard's Dairyman July 1995 p 470

[216] Gilot P; Limbourg B; Development of species-specific enzyme-linked Journal of Clinical Microbiology, 1994 32 (5): 1211-6 May

[217] Adams; Mycobacterium cell wall components induce the production of TNF alpha, IL-1, and IL-6 by bovine monocytes and the murine macrophage cell line RAW 246.7. Microb Pathog 1994 Jun.; 16 (6) :401-11.

[218] Cocito C., Paratuberculosis, Clin Micdrobiol Rev 1994 Jul;7(3) : 328-45

[219]Pavlik I; Occurrence, economic significance and diagnosis of paratuberculosis, Vet Med (Praha) 1994; 39 (8) :451-96.

[220] Cocito, C.. Gilot, P. Coene, M, DeKesel, M. Poupart, P Vannuffel, P. Paratuberculosis, Clini-cal Microbiology Reviews July 1994 p. 128-345.

[221] Collins MT; Herd prevalence and geographic distribution of, and risk factors for, bovine para-tuberculosis in Wisconsin. J Am Vet Med Assoc 1994 Feb. 15;204 (4) :636-41.

[222] Taylor, T.K., C.R. Wilks, and D.S. McQueen. Isolation of Mycobacterium paratuberculosis from the milk of cows with Johne's disease. Vet. Rec. 1981; 109:532-533

[223] Sweeney RW. Whitlock RH. Mycobacterium paratuberculosis cultured from milk and supramammary lymph nodes of infected asymptomatic cows. J Clin Microbiol 1992:30:166-71.

[224] Cocito C., Paratuberculosis, Clin Micdrobiol Rev 1994 Jul;7(3) : 328-45

[225] Dell'Isola B; Detection of Mycobacterium paratuberculosis by polymerase chain reaction in children with Crohn's disease. J Infect Dis 1994 Feb;169(2) : 449-51.

[226] Wall S; Identification of spheroplast-like agents isolated from tissues of patients with Crohn's disease and control tissues by polymerase chain reaction. J Clin Microbiol 1993 May; 31 (5) : 1241-5.

[227] Hermon-Taylor J. Causation of Crohn's disease: the impact of clusters. Gastroenterology 1993: 104:643-6.

[228] Sweeney RW; Whitlock RH; Buckley CL; Diagnosis of paratuberculosis in dairy cattle, American Journal of Veterinary Research; 1994 55 (7):905-9 Jul

[229] Collins, MT; Comparison of polymerase chain reaction tests and faecal culture for detecting Mycobacterium paratuberculosis in bovine faeces. Vet Microbiol 1993 Sept; 36(3-4) : 289-99.

[230] Sanderson JD; Mycobacterium paratuberculosis DNA in Crohn''s disease tissue. Gut 1992 Jul.; 33 (7) : 890-6.

[231] Vannuffel p; Dieterich C; Naerhuyzen B; Gilot P; and others; Occurrence, in Crohn's disease, of antibodies directed against a species specific recombinant polypeptide of Mycobacterium paratuberculosis. Clin Diagn Lab Immunol 1994 Mar; 1 (2) : 241-3.

[232] Sweeney RW; Mycobacterium paratuberculosis cultured from milk and supramammary lymph nodes of infected asymptomatic cows. J Clin Microbiol 1992 Jan ; 30 (1) : 166-71.

[233] Proceedings ninety-ninth Annual Meeting of the United States Animal Health Association , Report of the Committee on Johne's Disease, Reno Nevada, Oct 28, 1995, page 317-325.

[234] Proceedings ninety-ninth Annual Meeting of the United States Animal Health Association , Report of the Committee on Johne's Disease, Reno Nevada, Oct 28, 1995, page 317-325.

[235] Hoards Dairyman Jan 25, 1995

[236] Cocito C., Paratuberculosis, Clin Micdrobiol Rev 1994 Jul;7(3) : 328-45

[237] Montal, d; Indian J Exp Biol 1994 May; 32 (5): 318-23

[238] Collins, MT; Paratuberculosis and Crohn's Disease: a Relationship?, Proceedings ninty-eighth annual meeting of the United States Animal Health Association 1994.

MARBLE MOUNTAIN PUBLISHING
P.O. BOX 668
PHOENIX, OREGON 97535
FAX: 541- 488-5368  PHONE 541-482-2048

YES PLEASE SEND ME THE BOOK MAD COWS
AND MILKGATE.   ENCLOSED IS $20.00.  Send
check or money order or use your credit card. No
C.O.D.'s. Card number:_____
Visa_____ MC_____ Expiration date_____

SEND TO:_____
ADDRESS_____
CITY_____STATE_____
ZIP_____

MARBLE MOUNTAIN PUBLISHING
P.O. BOX 668
PHOENIX, OREGON 97535
FAX: 541- 488-5368  PHONE 541-482-2048

YES PLEASE SEND ME THE BOOK MAD COWS
AND MILKGATE.   ENCLOSED IS $20.00. Send
check or money order or use your credit card. No
C.O.D.'s. Card number:_____
Visa_____ MC_____ Expiration date_____

SEND TO:_____
ADDRESS_____
CITY_____STATE_____
ZIP_____